FROM THE TRENCHES

FROM THE TRENCHES

A Victim and Therapist Talk About Mind Control and Ritual Abuse

Wendy Hoffman and
Alison Miller

Routledge
Taylor & Francis Group
LONDON AND NEW YORK

First published 2015 by Karnac Books Ltd.

Published 2018 by Routledge
2 Park Square, Milton Park, Abingdon, Oxon OX14 4RN
711 Third Avenue, New York, NY 10017, USA

Routledge is an imprint of the Taylor & Francis Group, an informa business

British Library Cataloguing in Publication Data

A C.I.P. for this book is available from the British Library

ISBN 9781782206019 (pbk)

Edited, designed and produced by The Studio Publishing Services Ltd
www.publishingservicesuk.co.uk
email: studio@publishingservicesuk.co.uk

CONTENTS

SECTION VIII: ODES ABOUT MIND CONTROL
by Wendy Hoffman

Note

Some names and descriptions of perpetrators have been changed and disguised out of necessity.

Should anything suspicious happen to Wendy Hoffman or Alison Miller or her family, then all names and locations of perpetrators will be released.

For Philippa and Tim,
whose dedicated support has made all the difference

INTRODUCTION

Dear Reader,

Let us introduce ourselves. We are two old women in our seventies who are still laboring and fighting in the trenches of the psychological and spiritual war against the evils of mind control and ritual abuse.

Wendy Hoffman, LCSW-C, is an American licensed clinical social worker who, more importantly, was a victim of organized mind control and ritual abuse from birth. She lived most of her life with her brain segmented and partitioned into thousands of parts, each trained for a specific task by the mind controllers. Struggling to get free, she eventually found the way to access her dissociated memories and reunite her brain. She has written two memoirs about her life experiences, *The Enslaved Queen* (2014) and *White Witch in a Black Robe* (2016a), as well as *Forceps* (2016b) a book of poetry about the rebirth of her self.

Alison Miller, PhD, is a Canadian clinical psychologist who worked initially in child and family therapy and parent education but, since 1990, has worked with survivors of mind control and ritual abuse. She has written *Healing the Unimaginable: Treating Ritual Abuse and Mind Control* for therapists, and *Becoming Yourself: Overcoming Mind Control and Ritual Abuse* for survivors.

We connected initially as therapist and client, and worked very hard to undo Wendy's mind control. Over the past few years, as our knowledge and understanding of these evils have increased, we have each been writing small articles or essays on various topics connected with the battle we are fighting. We have gathered these essays together into this book, *From the Trenches*. Rather than having a logical development of ideas from chapter to chapter, this book has collected the essays into topical sections, ending with Wendy's odes to the different kinds of inner parts, some of who lived her mind-controlled life, and also live in other survivors' inner worlds.

You may read them in any order you wish. Some of these essays are directed primarily to survivors, others to therapists and support people. If you are inexperienced with the subject matter, you might want to read our other books first, since some of the material in this book is quite advanced and will make the most sense to someone who understands how mind control works and what atrocities the mind controllers perpetrate.

We want to encourage survivors to find their whole selves and not give in to the fears perpetrators put in them, therapists to brave the complexities and horrors of this challenging and fascinating work, and supporters to rally to help those who have been victimized from infancy for the misfortune of being born into the wrong family. Every time someone gets free or desires to be free, victims, their therapists and helpers make another tear, another slit in the membrane of the soul of evil. We are all in this together, and together we can bring this empire down. It may not be completed in this generation, but it has begun.

Wendy and Alison

Protest

Ella Wheeler Wilcox

To sin by silence, when we should protest,
Makes cowards out of men. The human race
Has climbed on protest. Had no voice been raised
Against injustice, ignorance, and lust,
The inquisition yet would serve the law,
And guillotines decide our least disputes.
The few who dare, must speak and speak again
To right the wrongs of many. Speech, thank God,
No vested power in this great day and land
Can gag or throttle. Press and voice may cry
Loud disapproval of existing ills;
May criticise oppression and condemn
The lawlessness of wealth-protecting laws
That let the children and childbearers toil
To purchase ease for idle millionaires.

Therefore I do protest against the boast
Of independence in this mighty land.
Call no chain strong, which holds one rusted link.
Call no land free, that holds one fettered slave.
Until the manacled slim wrists of babes
Are loosed to toss in childish sport and glee,
Until the mother bears no burden, save
The precious one beneath her heart, until
God's soil is rescued from the clutch of greed
And given back to labor, let no man
Call this the land of freedom.

SECTION I

UNDERSTANDING MIND CONTROL

A dozen myths therapists might believe

Alison Miller

Therapists with the usual kinds of training believe some myths that can impede their effectiveness in treating survivors of mind control and ritual abuse. Here are some I have heard.

1. *Myth*: *DID (dissociative identity disorder, which used to be called multiple personality disorder, MPD) is rare, if it exists at all.* The reality is it that it affects at least 1% of the population. And if you include the people whose hundreds or thousands of segregated and organized parts are hidden behind a deceptive front, it is probably a much greater number. Many more people have ego states from unhappy or frightening experiences and can be overcome by strong emotions or false beliefs without actually having DID. They do not have access to the original cause of those emotional states, so tend to blame them on the present.

2. *Myth*: *Hearing voices always indicates psychosis.* The term "schizophrenia" means "split mind," which means having a dissociative disorder rather than a brain disease. Historically, the two conditions became mixed up. Now we are aware that dissociative people, whom I shall call multiples, are survivors of severe childhood trauma, whereas genuine schizophrenics might well have a brain disease. Many people who hear voices are dissociative, and are hearing other

parts of themselves talking to them or to one another. Other people hear thoughts out loud in their heads. This does not mean they are psychotic. Hallucinations can be flashbacks of abuse, and apparent delusions can be beliefs implanted by perpetrators (See the section on Lies.) Many people who have dissociative disorders are misdiagnosed as schizophrenic, especially if they talk about demons, or Satan, or the CIA, or mind control. They are likely to be survivors of organized abuse, and might be trying to tell their story to people who just write them off as deluded.

3. *Myth*: *People who frequently change their mood and emotional state, their perceptions, and their attitudes suffer from bipolar disorder and/or attention deficit disorder and/or schizophrenia*. Before diagnosing someone with any disorder that requires chemical treatment, it is important to rule out dissociative disorders, the conditions in which someone has many, relatively independent, "selves." Apparent attention deficit disorder can also really be hypervigilance, someone who has been abused constantly looking around for danger. Apparent bipolar disorder, especially the rapid-cycling type, can really be dissociative switching as different parts come to the forefront.

4. *Myth*: *There are effective brief therapy methods, such as cognitive–behavioral therapy, which will cure survivors*. When a person is severely abused on a regular basis for his or her entire childhood, and usually beyond, it is dishonoring to the survivor to suggest that three or four, or even a dozen, sessions of some special technique will clear up all the effects of this abuse. Victims of mind control and ritual abuse have suffered more than any other group of victims that I have heard of. We rightly make a big fuss about post traumatic stress disorder in military veterans and victims of rape. But what about victims of complex trauma, including emotional abandonment, infant and ongoing torture, child prostitution, and forced perpetration for years on end? Let us not kid ourselves about brief magic cures. "Empirically validated therapies" are useful for single contained problems. Recovery from mind control and ritual abuse rightfully takes years.

5. *Myth*: *The front person ("host") in a dissociative individual is real and the others are not*. All parts of a person are parts of the same brain, whose electrical circuits were segregated by severe early trauma. The front person is just a part who is specialized for dealing with daily life, which means that this part knows little or nothing about the trauma

or the life of the other parts. The average multiple has a series of front people at different stages of life. They are no more real or unreal than the other parts. Front people often say that they feel unreal, because they are only a small part of a person.

6. *Myth*: *Therapists should always work just with the front person, not talk to the "alters."* Multiplicity cannot be resolved without communication with the inside parts who hold the memory narratives, body sensations, and feelings from the trauma. The front person is sometimes too fragile to handle knowing those memories, and, in any case, he or she cannot find out what happened without communicating with the inside parts. Therapy with just the front person will get nowhere, because symptoms such as anxiety and depression, flashbacks and nightmares arise mainly from the hidden parts.

7. *Myth*: *All ritual abusers are satanists.* Many different groups use mind control on children: extremist political groups, intelligence agencies, organized crime, child pornographers, and, yes, satanists. All these groups also attempt to control the general population via the media.

8. *Myth*: *Survivors do not have the ability to recognize whether their memories are real.* Perpetrator groups put a lot of effort into convincing their victims that the memories that pop up unbidden are imagination, or something they saw on television, or anything other than reality. They also put a lot of effort into convincing society that certain kinds of bad things do not really happen, so if someone believes they happened to him or her, that person must be deceived and be having "false memories," possibly suggested by a therapist.

The reality is that survivors have very real memories, but these include memories of deceptions such as simulated murder and people in costumes. They also have memories of being told, while under the influence of drugs, hypnosis, and torture, that something quite different happened. Perpetrator groups work hard to make sure that what survivors believe to be their memories are distorted. They disguise identities. They often tell their lies to child parts in adults, as well as to actual children, giving false interpretations of what happened, interpretations which the child or child part has to accept or face dire consequences. It is, therefore, a very difficult task for a survivor to put together the entirety of a memory accurately. It requires bringing together all the insiders who have any part of that memory, including the part where they were taught false interpretations.

Still, many survivors know from bodily sensations as well as emotions that they must have had such experiences, regardless of whether the general public believes them or mother says they are invented. The body does not lie. Survivors can be strong and persistent in sorting out reality from the distortions taught to them by the perpetrators.

9. *Myth*: *Ritual abuse survivors are overly concerned about holidays and special dates, and these do not really matter*. These dates matter most to survivors of abuse by ritualistic, usually satanic, cults. That is because these groups expect their victims to attend rituals on these dates, which include the victim's own and family members' birthdays as well as major Christian and pagan holidays. Sometimes, a survivor is actually safe, but even then he or she is likely to have flashbacks and nightmares of the abuse that happened on these dates. More often, the survivor is still in touch with family members and is expected to attend the rituals.

10. *Myth*: *Demons attached to, or inserted in, children are real and must be ousted*. While I recognize that we cannot say with certainty whether or not evil spiritual entities exist, I can say, with quite a bit of certainty, that the "demons" that are attached to, or inserted in, children by ritually abusing perpetrator groups are simply child parts of the person, split off by a combination of drugs, threats, torture, terror, and forced perpetration. I have been working with ritual abuse survivors for twenty-seven years, and I have never met a real demon, but I have met a considerable number of fake demons. I have had clients on whom exorcisms or deliverances were performed, and the result was that "demon" parts went into hiding out of fear, taking with them the memories which needed to be processed for healing. They were afraid to be known to me because of the fear that I might try to destroy them. I have heard of other cases where these parts became angry and punished the rest of the personality system. Would you not do that if someone tried to kick you out of the only society you knew?

11. *Myth*: *Most survivors are not currently harassed*. Perpetrator groups who deliberately create dissociative disorders in their victims are very concerned about keeping their criminal activities, such as rape, murder, child prostitution, and pornography, secret. If a survivor begins to remember and tell about things that the group wants kept secret, parts of the survivor report this to a group member, and harassment begins. There is re-abuse, along with serious threats

to the survivor, the person the survivor tells, and anyone the survivor loves. Harassment of survivors is very common, and might be life-long. Survivors tend to believe the threats, including those to therapists, so might not tell their therapists about what is happening in the present. It is important to realize that physical harm to a therapist is very rare, because it can compromise the group's security. Perpetrator groups prefer to remain hidden from therapists, and find ways to discredit effective therapists, such as inducing clients to sue them or making complaints to their licensing boards.

Therapists, pay attention to subtle changes in your clients. If a client is suddenly angry at you without cause, as in the example I give in "Therapists' responses to survivors" (later in this book), it could indicate that perpetrators are trying to turn him or her against you. If a survivor client has physical symptoms which do not appear to arise from a physical cause, he or she could have been beaten up and not remember it. These things could arise from cult-loyal parts of them doing their jobs, but if that is not the case, the next possibility is current harassment that they do not remember. Wendy had persistent ear pain, especially when she took a plane journey to a conference and when she flew to visit me. The doctors could not find the cause afterwards. She was unaware that she had been beaten up just before taking the journeys. Doctors do not look for adults' symptoms being caused by current abuse.

12. *Myth*: *Survivors of mind control and ritual abuse cannot recover.* This is what the perpetrators want them, and you, to believe. Yes, people whose brains have been subdivided from birth through horrific experiences will need to undergo a long journey of recovery. But they can recover, their minds can be whole again, and they can become the persons they choose to be. The younger they begin this process, the longer they will have to live their own lives.

Pieces of self

Wendy Hoffman

If you are going to have a brain that is smashed into pieces, your perpetrators have to start when you are young—in infancy or before. The first splits are usually done when you are about one month old or under. Perpetrators create thirteen distinct sections of the mind then, one after the other, sometimes without a pause. Jobs will be assigned to each division and extensive trainings will begin as the infant victim ages. They teach visual and aural cues to trigger the robotic parts the mind controllers created. Years later, the perpetrators might braid and twist together pieces from some of the thirteen columns, or "edifices," or "rivers" to be used for more complex and secret criminal tasks. Life does not improve as you age unless you achieve prolonged physical safety.

Your task, if you are a victim attempting to find your way through these mazes of torture and dissociation, is to find the very young infant parts, and the memories of the infant splits. Just acknowledging that these splits exist helps loosen the whole internal mind control structure.

As you get to know the older parts created to do horrendous jobs for no money or reward and without you knowing what you had done, as you begin to take in the reality of your life as a blind automaton, as you realize you have been only a mindless puppet with tight strings intact, you will find all that overwhelming. Despair can be great, anger greater. Plus sadness that you have not had a life you can call your own. Integration—when the divisions of the mind self-erase and you get to know your abused selves—usually occurs in waves. After the one or two tidal waves when most of the pieces of brain come together, you often find fail-safe measures. There is should-you-ever-integrate-programming. Mine was placed under layers of psychedelic plastic sheets. Here, my infamous mind controller sectioned off little pieces of my main role—that of being one of the Illuminati queens—and hid them "never to be found" under these toxic barricades.

First, you work either up the internal hierarchy to the leaders of the system or down the hierarchy to the tortured infants. These parts spontaneously meld together. There might be one or more tidal waves of coming together. Always be on the lookout for a section or sections you have not found yet. Huge drug and electrical walls separate internal sections. The sections of your mind weave and braid together. Even if you do not want one solid chunk of mind, it will happen. Roots gravitate to water. Birds copulate in the air. Our minds want to be whole. We were created to be whole. Nature is stronger than crime. We can go back to our evolutionary beginnings. We can become both a new person and who we were from the beginning, as if untampered with. Humans cannot fight nature. Humans cannot fight God. Our lives can be un-usurped.

Look for the little pieces of self that are hidden away even after the major integrations. Even if these parts seem dead, carry them home, no matter how heavy they are. Lug them down masonic steps, out of burning buildings, unlock prison gates, open freezer doors, rip open barricades. Have a joyous celebration of reunification. Now you are whole. Now you are you. No one took your soul away permanently. You are the more powerful.

How to talk with a multiple*

Alison Miller

We tend to assume other people are like ourselves, unless they are in some way visibly different. For example, when someone has a different skin color or a strong foreign accent, we are aware that they may be different. But when they look and sound the same as us, it is difficult for us to understand that they may be different in their background and way of thinking.

One of the kinds of people we often have difficulty understanding is the person with a dissociated identity, an identity split into many selves rather than a single one. This condition used to be called "multiple personalities." In this essay, I am using the term "multiple," because some of my clients who are multiple prefer it to the more general term "dissociative," which can have many meanings. Everyone dissociates to some extent—for example, many people dissociate certain emotions and never consciously feel them. Everyone also has different parts of the self, but most of the population is not multiple.

People who have been through severe childhood abuse or other trauma have often learned to handle life through several different

* Much of the material in this chapter was also in Chapter Three of *Healing the Unimaginable.*

"selves" rather than a single unified self. Becoming many selves rather than one is a biological process in the brain that results from severe early trauma, which is often life threatening. Becoming multiple is not something that the person chooses, and it cannot begin in adulthood, only in early childhood. It is not just a product of creative imagination. Although all these "selves" are really parts of one person, they may experience themselves and one another as separate people.

A multiple's experience of life is very different from that of someone who has never been multiple. For someone who has always been a single personality, it is difficult to understand how a person who is multiple thinks. Often relatives and friends of a multiple, as well as support people and even therapists and other professionals, are unclear about how to talk to such a person. Here are a few thoughts which might help you understand the people you know who have multiple, rather than single, identities.

Talking with a multiple is like talking with someone from another culture

Although a multiple might not be visibly different from anyone else, the way he or she thinks is incredibly different, at least as different as the way someone thinks who comes from a completely different culture. We do not (or, at least, we should not) blame people from other cultural backgrounds for being different from us and for not completely understanding our culture. It is important to treat a multiple person with dignity and respect, just as you would someone from a foreign culture whose values and customs you do not yet understand.

First of all, do not assume that a multiple is really like you. They may look the same, but they are different. The dominant culture is one of non-multiples, so multiples have learned to hide their multiplicity and imitate those of us who are have a single personality ("singletons"). But it is only an imitation. Survivors of the kind of enforced mind control addressed in this book are all multiple, whether or not they are aware of it. They are programmed to hide their multiplicity, as mind control depends on multiplicity, and the people who abused them to make them multiple do not want any visible signs of the abuse.

A person who has a single personality cannot become a multiple at will. It requires many severe early traumatic experiences (such as sexual abuse and/or torture) to make a person's brain put up the barriers which give them several or many identities. Survivors of childhood mind control usually have hundreds of separately trained parts. Similarly, a multiple cannot become a singleton until and unless the barriers between the parts of the self ("alter personalities" or inner selves) are removed. Those barriers were put up for a purpose, so that the child could survive the abuse (from the victim's perspective), and so that the child will not remember what happened (from the abusers' perspective.) People who are multiple cannot think like us, and we cannot think like them, but we can learn to understand one another with respect for our differences.

Once you recognize the multiple is different from you, it is important to ask him or her to be your teacher about being multiple. You cannot just guess about it; you have to ask. Those multiples who are aware of their condition are usually glad to be asked. They get very lonely because they are not understood by other people. Child personalities in adult bodies, for example, sometimes feel nobody else understands them or recognizes their existence. They often like to be known, recognized, and talked to as the age they feel they are rather than the age the body is. Although you must be careful with this—child parts are all different: some are shy and some are outgoing; some like attention and others hate it.

When you ask what it is like to be multiple, be careful not to treat the person as if she or he is a curiosity. I remember how embarrassed I felt on my first night as a student in India, when I got changed for bed in a university residence, and a crowd of young women gathered to stare at me to see whether I was the same color all over! Just because a person is different does not mean she is less than human. I did not like having to "perform" (for example, sing English hit parade songs) for other students in India, while they all giggled at me and talked about how cute I was. Similarly, multiples do not like having to "perform" (for example, let child parts come out) for the entertainment of singletons. They are people, too, and their human dignity is important.

For a multiple, being multiple is his or her normal state of mind. It is difficult for him or her to understand how singletons think, and he or she may think it is you who are strange. That is, if he or she even knows that you are not like him or her. I have met several multiples who just assume that everyone else "loses" periods of time (when another "front person" part is in charge of the body), finds themselves in places without knowing how they got there, and/or hears voices or audible thoughts inside their head.

We singletons are well adapted for living in safety, being conscious of everything that happens to us. A multiple is well adapted for living with ongoing trauma. I once heard a prison psychologist say he would not treat multiples in prison, because to survive well in prison you needed to be multiple, as prison is so traumatic. Even in normal life there are sometimes advantages to being multiple. I knew a multiple who had a part called "Brain" who memorized all her textbooks and was able to remember everything on exams word for word. I knew another who had parts with all kinds of special "idiot savant" abilities. When a part is able to focus on only one thing, without the distractions of emotions, everyday life, and other thoughts, he or she may be able to perform that task exceptionally well. Abuser groups use this to train parts in special skills such as memorizing information to deliver to politicians.

Just as you should not assume that someone from another culture should want to join your culture and give up his or her own, do not assume that a multiple wants to become a singleton. Some do, some do not. Many well-adapted multiples, whose parts cooperate well, prefer to stay as a community of coordinated selves rather than become a single self. They feel that they would be lonely without insiders to talk with. They forget, however, that many of those insiders are still in pain or trapped in horrible memories, and also that leaving programming untouched can put them in danger.

Talking with a multiple is like talking with people who change places undetectably

Imagine there are a number of identical brothers or sisters who impersonate one another. They are able to change places so fast that you cannot detect it, so fast that you may talk to many within one conversation. However, if you know them as individuals, you learn to recognize them not by their physical appearance but by their characteristic moods, tones of voice, facial expressions, and other body language. It is the same with alter personalities (parts) of multiples. They *look* the same, but they act differently. You may also see physical evidence of them changing places in eye movements, body tremors, losing track of conversation, and other subtle signs. Most multiples, however, do not show dramatic physical symptoms of "switching." Many (but not all) deliberately designed multiples have a "front" or "shell" part who is out all the time, along with other parts who change behind the shell. The shell part bridges the transitions smoothly so the individual does not appear multiple at all. However, such people sometimes have parts who can take over entirely, with the front part disappeared inside and unaware that time has been lost. The larger the number of parts, the less detectable will be the switches. And the more inner communication is established between the parts (usually through therapy), the easier will be the transitions between parts being "out" (in control of the body), since some may listen in on others' conversations in the world. Often, the only sign of a switch might be the body language of another part. Survivors of complex mind control may be trained to switch seamlessly and to sound like adults at all times, except when their external controllers call out hidden child parts for torture, training, or reporting. Others are designed to look "crazy" through constant switching.

One confusing thing about many multiples is that at one time they may completely know and believe that they are multiple, and at another time they may deny it completely. Most multiples have at least one "front person," whose purpose is to deal with the normal outside world and handle everyday normal life. When a child is being abused on an ongoing basis, he or she needs to be able to function even though the abuse is occurring. So, the child develops a "front person" (formerly known as the "host" personality, in contrast to the "alter" personalities) who is unaware of the abuse and also of the multiplicity. The term "host" is a misleading term, developed by singletons who assumed that the front person is more real or more important than the other parts. That is why I prefer "front person."

Sometimes there are several front people, each of whom assumes he or she is the real one and is amnestic for the existence of the others. Some front people have a great deal of difficulty accepting that they are multiple. The word "personalities" or "alters" might frighten them. Whether the person acknowledges that he or she is multiple, then, depends on who is "out" in conscious control of the body and on how much contact the front person has with the "inside world." Some multiples always have the front person present in everyday life and in therapy sessions, even when another part is in control of the behavior and feelings. These people are generally not diagnosed with dissociative identity disorder (DID), and do not "lose time" in the same way that those who are diagnosed with DID do, in the middle of a regular day. Some people used to be visibly multiple when they were young, but with maturity and a stable, safe life, have developed a strong person who handles all of present-day life. Many things are easier for such people than for DID multiples, because they do not lose time or find money has been spent on toys. However, it is easier for such a person than for someone with DID to assume that negative feelings are caused by present situations when they actually come from old traumas which have been triggered by something in the present. Parts with these feelings are often lurking just behind the front person. One such multiple described herself as having someone like a plastic lens in the front, with four chairs just behind it, and different people occupying those chairs at different times.

Multiples who have accepted their multiplicity often call their parts "people"; this is who they are to them. They are just as real to them as people on the outside. Other multiples, who are less aware of those on the inside, find "parts" or "inner children" more acceptable terms. Although the parts or "selves" feel themselves to be complete persons, each tends to have a specific function and most of them are, in a way, one-dimensional. Do not assume that the front personality is the "real" person and the other personalities are less real. A question such as, "Is this Jane, or one of the alters?" is very irritating to multiples, especially if it happens not to be Jane who is "out." The front person is just a part, often one with little power in the system, little memory of what happened, and limited energy or emotions. In my experience, multiples in whom there is one strong front person tend to be those who were abused or traumatized for only a brief period of time, usually outside the home. Their long period of safety allowed them to build a strong "outside world" personality, but they still have hidden split-off parts, who either come out only occasionally or never come out but influence their behavior and feelings from time to time. Do not assume that the front person is able to control the behavior of the other parts if he or she only "takes responsibility." If a multiple's front person tells you that someone inside wants to kill her, for example, she is telling you that she does not have control over it, and telling her to take control will not help.

Since parts change places a lot, you should not assume that the person you are talking to remembers what the body has seen, heard, done, or said, even five minutes ago. Amnesia is a major distinguishing characteristic of multiples, especially if they have DID. If the part who was "out" when something happened has "gone inside", the person will not remember what happened. Multiples learn to cover up for loss of time. It is common that a multiple who does not yet know he or she is multiple does not realize time has been lost, and will deny doing things he or she has been seen doing, leading to a reputation as a liar. When a multiple realizes that another part may have done it, he or she will often pretend to remember the incident to hide the time loss. However, the awareness may spur some on to delve into their minds and discover dissociation.

When meeting new inside parts, do not assume they are orientated in time and place. They often believe they are still living in the situation where the abuse occurred, or some other past time. Often, they do not know that the body has grown up. I find it helpful to have a newspaper or magazine with a recent date to show them the year, and to have a mirror so they can see what their body looks like now, though sometimes this is too great a shock for them if many years have gone by, and many multiples are afraid of mirrors because mirrors were used to deceive them.

Kinds of parts or personalities

Many, usually a majority, of the parts feel themselves to be children, so you should not assume you are talking to an adult at all times. There could be some who are too young to talk or to understand language. Although it is controversial among therapists who treat people with dissociated identities, I believe that child parts of a multiple split off during childhood, not later, and are still developmentally children. They are not "normal" children, however. The "happy" ones tend to deny negative reality and get themselves into abusive situations. The "unhappy" ones hold strong emotions such as fear and anger. Child parts are often concrete and literal in their thought processes and awkward with their bodies, and might hold superstitious childish beliefs, communicated to them by abusers during the person's actual childhood. I have had the experience of an adult woman sitting on the floor and putting out her feet for me to tie her shoes, assuming she was in preschool. I have been with an adult man when he stood on his head on my office couch, because the child that he "was" at that moment preferred that position. I have been with adults whose "out" personalities knew no English, but spoke languages the person had learned in early childhood and then forgotten. I have had a woman fall down my office stairs because a baby part who did not know how to walk came "out" at the top of the stairs. (After that, I started making home visits to her.)

Some therapists who work with dissociative disorders believe that child parts are actually adults' conceptions of what children are like, rather than actual children. I do not believe this myself, but I do believe that a part who says he or she is older than the body is not really older, but is a child's, or a young adult's, conception of an older person. And an opposite-sex part (a male in a female body, for instance) is more like a young girl's idea of what a boy is like than like a real boy. Boys in women's bodies usually represent the part of the person who has traits that are traditionally considered masculine, such as bravery or anger; girls in men's bodies often have supposedly "feminine" traits such as fear. It is not worth arguing with parts about whether they really are what they believe they are. It is more important to treat the whole person with respect, in whatever aspect he or she presents to you (though it is important for all parts eventually to learn that they share a single body in the real world). The person had very important reasons for making parts the way they are. For example, a part may be a boy because boys do not have vaginas so he cannot be vaginally raped.

Some parts experience themselves as blind or deaf or mute, often as a result of a literal response to their abusers ("Do not talk about this" or "Do not look"). Some are "copy" parts (the technical term is "introjects") who believe they are someone else entirely; for example, a relative or an abuser. Do not deny the experience of any part. Each genuinely believes it is the person's mother, or a person of the opposite sex, or a dog, even though they are mistaken.

Some multiples have parts who think they are supernatural beings, such as demons. If they say this, they are mistaken. Often a child who has been shamed, verbally abused, and told they are evil, or made to do evil things by an abuser, can believe him or herself to be a demon. Some perpetrator groups actually tell child parts they are demons or devils or ghosts. Trying to exorcise "demon" parts of a person will only hinder their progress. Such parts need to be cared for like any child, and the responsibility for their abuse given back to the abusers rather than to any part of the child.

It is important to realize that parts have separate memories, feelings, and approaches to life, and do not necessarily know what the other parts do or think, even though they are actually all parts of one person. Each part, including the front person, is very limited. Although he or she has a sense of separate identity and agency, he or she is unable to feel some emotions or engage in some behaviors. Many parts, especially front people, feel hollow, depersonalized, or uncertain of their identity, precisely because they *are* just part of a whole. Nevertheless, they and others in the system experience them as separate (wounded) people.

Multiples and responsibility

Alter personalities (parts) hold memories only of the experiences in the person's life which those parts have actually lived. One part cannot be held responsible for events they actually do not remember or had no control over. I once treated a ten-year-old girl who had just one inner part in addition to the main person, a three-year-old with the same name as her. When she got bored in school, the ten-year-old would "go inside" her head, and the three-year-old would come "out" into the body and behave like a three-year-old, which was inappropriate for the classroom. The ten-year-old would then find herself in the school office in trouble with the principal, without any idea of what had happened. While the whole person could be said to be responsible for the behavior, the ten-year-old was not, and the three-year-old was too young to realize what was wrong with her behavior. Sometimes, when an inappropriate behavior happens, the front person just does not know about it, and is only aware of "lost time." At other times, the front person may be conscious of what is happening but unable to control it.

Be especially careful about assigning responsibility and blame—the part you are talking to may not be responsible for a behavior or even know about it. Most multiples have been abused emotionally as well as (usually) physically and sexually, and are very sensitive to blame. The whole story of their lives in the "outside" world is of being held responsible for things they do not remember doing. They are accused of lying and manipulating. They might, at times, lie and manipulate, especially when parts are out who are very young or who cannot feel pain or cannot feel guilt. But much of the time they just do not know what happened, or know but had no control over it.

If you want to deal with issues of responsibility, find and talk with the part who is actually responsible. This may be either the part who performed the behavior, or another part who made him or her do it. Remember to be gentle even with the part who is responsible. People who lie and manipulate, whether or not they are multiple, have usually learned to do this because of living with severe punishment. It takes experience in a safe world to learn more direct strategies of getting needs met.

Talking with a multiple is like talking on the phone with a group of housemates

Although only one part at a time can control the multiple's voice and actually talk with you, many can hear you and can send messages to you. Talking to a multiple is like being on the phone to someone in a large house. Only one person at a time is able to speak to you but the house phone has a speaker which broadcasts your words to others in the vicinity, so that they can hear you and can speak to the one on the phone and send messages to you. The person who was on the phone a minute ago may be nearby listening or may be completely out of the room. Those outside the range of the speaker cannot hear you, but someone can be sent to get them.

Do assume that some others inside can hear you even when one part is on the outside, or can be sent a message. This applies even when the presenting part is deaf, catatonic, or a baby. You can talk through the presenting part to others in the system. Not everyone can hear you, but many, especially the important ones, can. Especially with a mind-controlled multiple, the important parts are always listening in order to guard the person's safety and the perpetrator group's security in the outside world.

When multiples begin therapy, they often do not have very good internal communication. It is important to assist them in improving this communication. I frequently ask other parts to speak to the one on the "phone" to me, letting this one know the answer to some question I asked. For example, when a part was grieving because she did not remember what her dead mother looked like, I asked the others listening to give her a picture of her mother, and she not only saw a picture, she heard her mother's voice. I encourage the one on the "phone" (talking with me) to "ask inside" to the others and get to know them. I respect the ones who come out spontaneously to talk with me, but I also ask to speak to others, and if they will not (or are not permitted to) speak to me directly, then I ask that messages be relayed back and forth to them.

Talking with a multiple is talking with someone who has been badly abused

Although DID stands for "dissociative identity disorder," I regard it as mental injury rather than mental illness. The way a person becomes multiple is through severe and prolonged early trauma, usually child abuse. Many of the parts of a multiple have known nothing but abuse. So they will expect you to abuse them, since they assume this is the normal state of affairs. I remember informing one seductive child part that I was not going to have sex with her. She responded indignantly, "Why not? That's what kids are *for*." Other parts have cowered, waiting for me to hit them, or been afraid to look up lest I look scary, or waited suspiciously for my next move.

Many multiples have lived with people who were themselves multiple, and changed unexpectedly from warm and loving to cruel and abusive. They will expect you to change in this way, and only time will prove to them that you do not. Do not take a multiple's negative expectations personally. Be consistently warm and respectful, and keep your promises, so that parts can learn to trust you. It is also important to take responsibility and apologize for your mistakes, so that the multiple's true experience of your mistakes is validated, and he or she learns the difference between mistakes and deliberate cruelty. Most multiples have been severely punished for making mistakes, and the example of someone who can acknowledge her or his own mistakes without dwelling on them is a healthy one for them.

Do not ever tell a multiple to "grow up." One teenage multiple who became my client spent a long time with a previous therapist until finally a young part gained the courage to come out and sit at the therapist's feet. The therapist told her to grow up and act her age. It was devastating to her, and prevented any disclosure of what had happened to her.

Do not ever tell a multiple to "forget the past." The past did unbelievably serious damage to the person, so much damage that parts of him or her are still stuck in childhood and are unable to grow up without help. Non-multiples often assume that the front person is able to control the behavior and feelings of the other parts, and is "living in the past" by "allowing" them to exist. This just is not true. The dissociation that split off the parts happened as a physiological process in early childhood, and cannot be dropped at will. The front person is often one of the least powerful parts in the system.

There is a difference between spontaneous multiplicity and deliberately designed multiplicity. Organized perpetrator groups use drugs, electricity, and torture to create the kind of personality system they want. People abused by these groups may have a set of parts created by abuse at home, but they also have complicated organized personality systems.

Talking with a multiple is like talking with a family whose members usually do not get along

Do not expect the person who is multiple to be consistent or to have internal harmony. At the start of therapy, most multiples have internal battles for control. The front person often has little or no control over switching. The parts may fight to be "out", or may push others "out" in order to stay inside. Decision-making is difficult, and decisions made by one part will be reversed by another, until internal communication and problem-solving have been learned. Simple things like shopping or eating can become incredibly difficult. Other survivors are, at least apparently, high functioning.

Democratic decision-making is not usually learned in the childhood of a multiple. Their families are typically arbitrary dictatorships, in which adults demand that they constantly obey out of fear of punishment, even when the rules are inconsistent. It is not, therefore, surprising that, until the person has been in the recovery process some time, parts often cannot agree on decisions. That is the nature of multiplicity. "Eww, Jane got us dressed this morning," or "I do not like her having sex with *my* body" are typical comments of parts about one another. They will often express anger and even hatred for one another. It is hard for them to realize that they all represent legitimate parts of one person, and to respect how each part helped the person survive the extreme situation in which they grew up.

Helping a multiple

The very things which helped the person as a child survive extreme trauma now get in the way of their effective living as an adult. If a child has to live with carers who hurt her, and cannot escape it, it is better for her not to know it some of the time. But when she is an adult, it does not work very well for her not to remember some of what happens in her everyday life. It does not work very well for her to have different inside "people" make opposite decisions for her life, and reverse one another's decisions, spend her money on things that different parts of her would never buy, take her places that other parts of her would never go, and so on. If an adult is still being abused, it is better for that person to have conscious awareness of it so he or she can decide what to do about it.

Those of us who were more fortunate in our early experiences can help the parts of the multiples we know to learn about love, trust, and cooperation. We can do this by being loving, trustworthy, and cooperative.

A first step in teaching cooperation is to be careful not to show favoritism among parts. Every part is there for a purpose, and is an important part of the system. Most hostile parts are using anger to protect vulnerable parts inside, usually young children. Do not be afraid of hostile parts. "Every persecutor is a misguided protector." Acknowledge that they are protectors, and offer to work with them to improve their, and your, ability to protect the client and the hurt parts. Especially in ritually abused clients, hostile parts (including demons) often turn out to be young children. If they seem dangerous, talk with them at first through another part. But do not act scared, or it will be a self-fulfilling prophecy. If you like all parts, it will help them learn to like and accept one another.

Help them "talk inside." Although talking internally may seem to make the person "more" multiple, in that they will hear voices and become aware of more parts, it will actually improve communication between the front person and the other parts, and the long-term result will be that they will become better organized and work more like an integrated person. The goal is "co-consciousness," with whichever part is "out" in the body being aware of the needs and viewpoints of all the other parts, so that effective decisions can be made by the whole person rather than by just one part at a time.

Do not talk too much about integration or fusion between parts, especially at the start. In many cases, parts are afraid that if this happens they will die. It works better to talk about walls between "inside people" no longer being needed than about the "people" disappearing or merging. Respect their choice not to fuse until and unless they are ready. My experience is that as parts share experiences and memories, the walls between them dissolve, either gradually (when they are co-conscious much of the time) or suddenly (during a major piece of memory work), and the integration naturally happens when they are ready. Not all survivors will be capable of integration, and it can be dangerous to insist on it. It takes inordinate strength to tolerate awareness of all of a life of horrendous abuse.

Imposed internal and political structures

Wendy Hoffman

As soon as children have any capacity to understand shapes, their programmers begin to install imagined geometric structures within them. Different groups use different structures and arrange and layer them in specific ways. I can only talk about the one installed in me, which started out as a pyramid or triangle. Although other survivors may have different structures, they may have similar sections and types of training since these groups employ proven formulas for mind control. Perpetrators record most mind control interventions in official books that are now computerized.

The programmers show a small child a physical representation of the geometric shape that they plan to use, and tell that child to imagine that shape inside his or her mind. This shape will be the centerpiece of the internal structure within which the various mind-controlled parts of the person will be lodged. Programmers will add other shapes in various sizes and orientations later, but the first shape is usually most dominant.

My central pyramid was right side up and divided into five horizontal sections. The first installed section was the Kaballah, a corruption of the authentic Kaballah. Originally known as the "tree of life," the real Kaballah is a mystical religion that aspires for purity. Those groups that hijack this ancient philosophy turn it on its head and render it a means for achieving evil. Here it breathes its beliefs into the whole interior system. The Kaballah tree has branches that extend throughout the body and life, and its many leaves hold numerous divisions and programs.

If the child-victim is one of those who is designated to have the Kaballah system installed, when the mind control begins, the programmer tortures the infant-victim until thirteen personalities or brain splits are achieved. Each split in the infant is assigned a color and a letter (mine were in a foreign language) and (in my case, at least) given a doll representing it as an internal "person." Each doll was placed in a container on the bumper guard of my crib. These original parts become the basis for future mind control. The basic structure of the infant's fractured mind becomes cemented about a year or two after these initial splits.

The Kaballah tree has branches which are represented as pathways, and in their hidden cult life, children are forced to walk along pathways which represent these branches. During these pathway trainings, the leaders traumatize the toddler or child to teach lies such as that the child will never escape, is worthless, will always be watched, and that they belong with these cult members and not with regular people in the outside world. This constitutes the Kaballah foundation. All its training is torture-based.

In my internal structure, the next lower level going upward toward the apex of the pyramid was Luciferianism. This sub-religion permeated my whole structure. These cults, including some Masonic groups, worship Lucifer. Little distinction exists between Lucifer and Satan, though Satan is represented more in nature and Lucifer in politics. Perpetrators and unwilling members can come from two groups. Luciferianism is usually one of the groups dominating people from multiple groups of this criminal world.

Within the pyramid, next came the Illuminati, with deep roots in the Kaballah groups. The Illuminati use multiple innocuous names for themselves such as "Pinnacle of Small Changes" or "Movement of Small Increases." These titles disguise its ruthless ambition to conquer and dominate the world. I'll use the commonplace term 'Illuminati' in this essay even though this popular term is not how the original group identifies themselves.

On top of that horizontal division was MKUltra, indicating secret experiments in mind control. The perpetrators who created this division steal children's minds and render them unknowing slaves who perform roles that corrupt governments need for their continuation in power. People continue these hidden crimes today. This group has no overt religious affiliations.

The apex of this pyramid within my internal system was Nazism. I am writing primarily about western "democracies" and their groups vying for supremacy, because that is the part of the world I was trained in. In my memoir *White Witch in a Black Robe,* I write that the racism this group is known for is a golden apple thrown out to distract the angry masses from its real purpose. Like the Illuminati members, the Nazi group wants to conquer and control the world. Nazism is in competition with the Illuminati, sometimes one or the other being in power politically. People would be amazed how many twenty-first century Nazis exist. Many look like ordinary people, some even show leftist leanings. When some of the cruder members slip into their Nazi personas and drop their masks, they stalk about in a bullying way as their true natures are exposed. Some people belonging to minority groups have been coerced into working for Nazis. Both the Nazis and the Illuminati worship Lucifer (even if some of their leaders don't believe in the religion). Traditional organized crime (called the Mafia, although it is not necessarily Italian) with its money-making demands for child prostitution and pornography, smuggling illegal goods and drugs, stealing babies, mounting animal fights and other crimes, were located in the Nazi section of my internal structure and were conducted by people connected with the Nazis in my life. Depending on which group has political ascendancy in a particular country, that section of mind-controlled people's inner structures will be placed above the section created by other groups.

The programmers who inserted the right-side up pyramid internally could also turn it upside down to reflect external politics. That means that sometimes the Illuminati with its roots planted in the Kaballah group would be higher, and sometimes the Nazi would rule internally and in the world. Both the Illuminati and Nazi groups believe they have the right to impose such a structure on the universe. We see this push and pull in world politics as at least the developed world becomes steadily more satanic. The stereotype of a few hidden individuals making decisions and ruling the world is an accurate portrayal. Sometimes persons who are hidden Illuminati leaders rule, and at other times those who are hidden Nazi leaders rule. This tug of war shows in political elections, even recent ones. The groups vie with each other. Each group wants exclusive power. But they are all Luciferians the way denominations of other religions are still under the same umbrella, and they often work together.

All the groups consider a mind controlled person a worthwhile specimen to own, and they secretly steal from one another. One group can plant parts with codes and triggers in victims' minds, and other groups may suspect something, but won't be able to find them. These thefts are not recorded in the victims' general records but only in the records of the group that conducted the theft.

There is a boom of conspiracy theories, as people try to figure out what is behind frightening global events. Few people realize that these satanic groups order assassinations. Isolated and unattached assassins are rare, if they exist at all. Many if not most of the political assassinations are from one of these groups fighting the other, using mind-controlled people as assassins. The conspiracy theorists, who are often good-hearted people who try but can't conceive of the extent of human evil, get that wrong, and the people who know through experience are unable to provide proof.

Who an infant born into these groups will become and how they will be used are set in its earliest days of life. There are no choices. Only mind control.

What countries become depends on which group's candidate wins an election with a pre-arranged agreement of who will win. It seems pre-arranged by hidden rulers and the groups appear to take turns, though not in a neat order. On occasion, a candidate without satanic affiliations runs in an election. That candidate will either be persuaded to withdraw or will lose, sometimes by a small margin. Citizens are looking for change and a better way, but Illuminati and Nazis don't want to give up their grip. And people adamantly don't want to hear this truth. Their resistance makes it easy for the criminal groups. Some people notice that the wealthy have entitlements but not the poor, or that the climate has changed and the environment is perhaps permanently spoiled, but they don't want to know the true nature of their elected officials. If a government official who is from satanism appears to do something right, it will be a matter of throwing the masses a crumb. Rulers from satanism do not mean to do good.

Even though some important world leaders are satanists, it doesn't follow that they have permanently won this battle. People can still object, rebel and protest. Even if leaders have sold out, the world is not forever lost. There are far fewer satanists than ordinary life people. Courageous citizens of the normal world can rise up and demand safety and justice.

Hand signals

Wendy Hoffman

After those who are chosen to be victims of mind control have just been born, perpetrators immediately begin fluttering their hands in the infants' faces. Of course, the infant victims have no idea what the hand movements signify. The programmers are sensitizing the babies to hand motions and teaching them to watch hands closely.

By the time these babies are toddlers, perpetrators begin to attach assigned meanings to the movements. Over time, the children learn the specific hand sequence to sit, go, lie down, fall asleep, be quiet, run, leave, enter, drop the evidence, hide something in specific places, such as under the steps, deny, murder, shoot, kidnap, steal, poison, drop a pill in a drink, forget everything, or remember nothing. Each one has its own configuration of fingers, wrist motions and right- or left-handedness. Parts of the person can be called out by pressure on the victim's left shoulder. A hand signal coupled with a visual cue or sound is sufficient for a trained, programmed assassin part of a person to perform a murder in public, and I believe this has happened.

Before I began my authentic recovery and was still thwarted by close-down specialists, something occurred that stunned me. I was a graduate student studying social work. My field placement was in

Harlem. I led a group of parents who had lost their children to government agencies, addicts trying hard, or not so hard, to stop drinking and drugging, and people straight from the ghettoes who had few, if any, social advantages. We explored the outside world. We made trips to the library, which most had never visited, walked around the neighborhood, talked about the emotional issues plaguing their lives. Our bonds became closer. At the end of the term, I had to leave because I was a student. They gave a party for me on the last day, paying for refreshments with their own meager money. This would be our last time together and was a tender time for us all. During the party, a secretary stood in the doorway, called my name and simultaneously motioned with the middle finger of her left hand. Had she used her right finger, I would not have risen like a mindless robot and left the room. Had she not innocently combined my name with the hand movement, I would not have had a hidden part emerge, obeying what some inside child part thought was a handler's order. By the time I came out of my trance, the members of my group had dissipated. I missed out on my last goodbye and they missed out on all of my gratitude. I did not consciously know yet of all the mind-controlled parts inside me. I had not yet met the several thousands of them, but I knew then that something was terribly wrong with me and that I was vulnerable to any wind, that I was not my own person.

When people who have been mind-controlled begin their journey into knowledge, they are often afraid to go outside because they fear hand signals. At survivors' conferences about mind control, victims are sent to give vulnerable speakers and participants hand signals. An administrator might ask the audience to cease using hand signals and, as happened at a recent conference, many in the audience persist in trying to trigger people. One older woman claimed she had a skin problem that made her scratch her face repeatedly. That seemed like a reasonable explanation and people felt sympathy for her. However, during a break in the conference talks, she sought me out, switched, and performed elaborate hand signals inches from my nose. Her programmed hand signals meant that I belonged to the cult and should return. Some of the hand signals meant that I should commit suicide. Most of the people using their hands in this way do not know what they are doing. Their front person is oblivious and the parts of them performing these actions are responding to programmed commands.

Perpetrator groups are serious about making their victims sensitive to responding to hand signals and also accomplished in demonstrating these signals to others. Perpetrators can, thereby, control people in public without saying a word. They also teach and practice foot signals and many other visual cues. Some groups are more intent on using hand signals than others. For example, the ritually abusing group of Masons use them extensively but most perpetrator groups rely on them to some degree.

Survivors who received hand signal trainings cannot be fully free until they associate how they were trained to respond to, and give, hand signals. This remembering is a giant step toward not being an automaton, and it makes going out in public safer. When someone makes a deliberate hand signal in my face now, the muscles around my brain tense and my mind slides into a memory of when that signal was programmed into my brain. I am then not vulnerable to it.

At times, it can be helpful to use a hand signal to avoid danger. When I was working as a therapist, a client stood up during a therapy session and advanced toward me with her arms and hands out. It was clear to me that she intended to strangle me, not because she wanted to, but because she had been given instructions to do so. I did a hand signal back to her, and she switched and took her seat.

Disinformation*

Alison Miller

Today, I looked at the description of yet another book about mind control and ritual abuse, purporting to describe what really goes on and offering a cure. Books, websites, YouTube videos, speakers at conferences, you name it—plenty of information is out there. But how do you tell the difference between genuinely helpful information and disinformation, which means information that purports to be true but is designed to mislead you?

The trick with disinformation is to include lots of correct information. However, that correct information consists of things that are already known, so the writer is not revealing anything new. When you have become hooked on reading the writing of someone who seems to know the truth, you suddenly discover that the truth you know has been mixed with something you have not heard before, which might, on first reading, seem utterly outrageous, such as "All ritual abuse and mind control is being managed at the highest level by aliens," or "The cult is breeding half-human, half-animal creatures [chimeras] and keeps them in secret underground locations." Besides disinformation

* A version of this chapter was published in the online journal *Survivorship*, Summer 2017.

about what the abusers do, there is disinformation about the healing process, such as "The true subconscious can instantly heal all the parts if they just say they want healing," or "The way to resolve dissociated traumatic memories is to just avoid the negative and focus instead on the details of positive memories," or "If you rebalance your body's energies, you will be healed."

In order to sort out truth from deliberately planted fiction, you need to engage your critical thinking skills. A philosophy web page (http://philosophy.hku.hk/think/criticalct.php) defines critical thinking as "the ability to think clearly and rationally about what to do or what to believe. It includes the ability to engage in reflective and independent thinking, and includes understanding the logical connections between ideas, evaluating arguments, and detecting inconsistencies and mistakes in reasoning." These are skills the abuser group did *not* want you to develop. They wanted you to believe what they said and obey them without questioning. Learning critical thinking is an important part of recovery.

Let us apply critical thinking skills to the examples I gave above from disinformation sources. "All ritual abuse and mind control are being managed at the highest level by aliens." Some versions of this one involve human-sized lizard-like creatures, others the gray aliens we see in abduction stories. I have been a reader of science fiction since I was about fourteen, and one thing I have learned is that creatures from other planets would not be two-legged and two-armed creatures like us, or like the lizards and grays. Genuine aliens might well breathe other gases than oxygen and have different shapes from any living earthly creatures (see the film *Arrival* for an example.) However, human beings could easily put on the kind of rubber masks you can buy around Halloween in order to look like aliens. Which is more likely?

How about "The cult is breeding half-human, half-animal creatures and keeps them in secret underground locations?" You cannot disprove this. However, I know (because my son is a researcher on the human genome in the world's leading university for this subject) that genomics has not advanced anywhere near the point where something like this could be done, and this would hold true even if there were secret cult or government research somewhere else. The speaker I heard on this topic believed she had given birth to such beings and was communicating with them telepathically. She was very sincere.

Very sincerely deluded. When I spoke with another ritual abuse survivor who had an inside part who believed itself to be a chimera, I investigated a little more and discovered it was a young girl who could run fast and was told she was half horse. As for the speaker who heard her "children" telepathically, my logical thinking tells me that the voices she heard were probably dissociated child parts of herself who had been told they were her children and were chimeras.

Another purpose of disinformation is to make the general public, including therapists, believe that if they think ritual abuse or mind control is real, they also have to believe in things they find completely impossible, such as some of the more outrageous claims made by the disinformation websites. So they dismiss the truth along with the falsehoods.

What about the healing methods that might be disinformation? As a survivor, you are hungry for anything that will help relieve your distress, especially if it is quick and easy rather than requiring you to work through what really happened to you. So you seize upon the correct descriptions of your experiences, and then think that if the author was able to describe what happened to you, he or she must be offering a correct understanding and proposal for cure. But this is not so.

Perpetrator groups are very eager to divert survivors away from anything which will genuinely help them heal, as healing will involve discovering what happened to them and even why it happened. These are secrets the perpetrator groups guard closely. The disinformation books and websites are meant for you to discover and share with other survivors, and they will lead you away from the truths you do not yet know, not towards them.

"The true subconscious can instantly heal all the parts if they just say they want healing." Apply your critical thinking skills and say "I wish," but know it will not happen. This one seems a bit more plausible: "The way to resolve dissociated traumatic memories is to just avoid the negative and focus instead on the details of positive memories." There are plenty of therapists who try to do this. If you have had such a therapist, you may be aware of whether or not it actually works. Many mind control and ritual abuse survivors have to struggle very hard to come up with any positive memory, and might end up inventing one to please such a therapist. Finally, "If you rebalance your body's energies you will be healed." This requires moving your body in certain ways and allowing someone to touch your body. Such new approaches are currently quite popular, and have replaced the Christian "deliverances" as the favorite of cult-involved therapists. Be very careful about this: body movements and touches and signals can actually set off programming in survivors. Some "energy therapists" are very sincere and accidentally do this; others work for the bad guys, and what they do will close down your personality system and prevent you from healing.

Apply your critical thinking. Years of research have shown that the way to resolve dissociated traumatic memories is, first, to develop communication with your inside parts, and second, to put the traumatic memories together. See http://www.isst-d.org/default.asp?contentID=49, which are the guidelines for therapists put out by the International Society for the Study of Trauma and Dissociation. Every survivor would like to find a solution that did not involve getting near the horrific content and overwhelming negative feelings of the traumatic memories. It is tempting to jump at the chance of an easy and positive way of healing. Unfortunately, it does not work, and anyone who tells you it works is either misled or trying to mislead you. It might even cripple you.

When you go online, or purchase books, or attend conferences teaching about mind control and ritual abuse, keep your critical thinking abilities in the forefront of your mind. You can learn to distinguish between information and disinformation.

The choice

Wendy Hoffman

My therapist and intelligent, informed friends who know about this field have told me for years that I am not responsible for what cult perpetrators do. "They did that, not you," they say. Of course, I do not believe them. It just did not sink in or I would not let it sink in even after I heard it multiple times. Media messages sink in after two exposures, sometimes three, but I just could not receive that all this evil was not my fault. Ridiculous, I know.

Then one day, by chance, I read an interview with the Iranian Shirin Ebadi in the March 2016 issue of *TIME Magazine*. Even non-skeptical people realize that all forms of popular media are now controlled by criminal groups who distort the news and give us false messages. So it is particularly ironic and strange that a turning point for me came from a typical popular media publication. The interviewer asked the Nobel Peace Prize winner, whose family suffered because of her quest for freedom and justice and whose colleagues were jailed, whether she felt responsible for the prison sentences that followed her revolutionary work. She answered it was not she who harassed the victims, but the government. "It's the Iranian government that has to feel the guilt," she says ("13 Questions with Shirin Ebadi," March 17, 2016). Something clicked in my fragmented brain.

The credit goes to my therapist and friends who coached my thinking for years. The lawyer's comment was the tipping point.

I had escaped from my criminal group. Probably the leaders punished people I loved and had to leave behind unwillingly, just as they had with Ebadi. It is not I who tortured them. It is the criminal group. My heart is finally absorbing this lucidity.

I have a small garden behind my new home. Being a city person, it is a novelty for me. I did not even know what slugs and snails were, though I knew that snails are considered a French delicacy. At first I mistook the slimy slugs for my dog's feces. Experienced gardeners told me how to eradicate them. Put out shallow containers of beer. Sprinkle salt on them. I could not use the chemical poisons because of my dog. I also had tall, elegant lupin plants in my garden. The slugs and snails destroyed them and others. I had to cut everything back. I experimented with the recommended means of death. The beer worked in the beginning, but then the network of insect communication must have tipped newcomers off. I only found bits of leaves in the beer. I preferred the salt. The snails went back into their portable homes and the slugs shriveled to look like fetuses. The insects shrank into themselves the way I did when I was tortured. Like me, they looked for a place where only they could reside no matter what happened to their bodies. I noticed that baby snails and slugs fought harder than the grown-ups. One day, my soul rebelled. I asked myself what am I doing? I asked myself, why does my lupin have more of a right to life than the preying insects? The lupin is gorgeous, the insects disgusting to me, but who am I to choose one over the other?

The criminal leaders and experts evaluate their members whom they consider their property when they are infants and young children. The evaluators are looking to see what will motivate each individual. One aspect of the evaluation is to see which of these brand new human beings will place their own survival above others', and which will place others' survival above their own. The groups feel that is an important distinction. Their methodology is to threaten and terrorize each child. "Do this or we will kill him," they say. "Do this or we will skin him alive." Some children will do anything to spare another's life. That spared life could be a loved one's or not. It could belong to a stranger. Perpetrators can threaten to bomb the whole world, and these sensitive ones would sacrifice themselves to that lie also. As we saw in Alison's essay, children believe lies.

Some children put themselves first. They might not want their family and friends skinned alive and murdered, but mostly they do not want to be hurt themselves. They have to be manipulated in a different way. Usually, they are bribed. "Do this and we will give you that," evaluators say. Everything is for self-aggrandisement. They become the people who are given the important, well-paying jobs in society even though they are often not particularly competent and not equipped to be leaders.

This assessment period is short-lived. Children show their deeper natures fast. A normal person told me that children growing up in normal environments take much longer to find this preference out about themselves. They go through developmental stages and finally choose how they want to live. Cult children are born onto a battlefield. They have no childhoods. They make adult-type decisions as infants. They are a different kind of person.

Executioners use small cult children's hands to perform the slaughters during rituals and organized killing events. The executioners usually wear massive black leather gloves for their effect, insert the ritual knife into the child's hands and cover the child's hands with their own. "It's your fault we had to kill this person." "It's your fault we had to kill this animal." The animal is often a beloved pet. These lies will fill the first kind of child with unbearable guilt and grief. The second type of child will also despair and come to look for ways to build him or herself up. Neither type of child is particularly resilient after extreme trauma and will most likely carry these traumas throughout life.

Whether people put themselves or other people first is not caused by their being born into this kind of cult. The tendency may be genetic and from other early environmental influences. The preference has nothing to do with intelligence, analytic ability, creativity, or education. It is a primal tendency closely linked to survival—either the survival of the soul or of the body. People with no connections to criminal perpetrators eventually display the same distinctions. When the sensitive children realize they have done something wrong, they can become suicidal. When the self-important ones become agitated, they might have homicidal ideation.

I was controlled for the vast majority of my life by the fear of causing others to be hurt. I lost the one boy who loved me when I was four and a half. I do not cry easily, but I still cry when I think of him, almost seventy years later. I lost all my children, one after the other, but the inside part who lost one of my eight children did not know about the others. Each mother was isolated and uninformed, even though we all shared the same body. So I engaged in the same mistaken thinking time and time again, wanting to save a child. Finally, because I had some help, I extricated myself from my desire to try to save my adult child and left my grandchildren, too. It was difficult to leave them all, even though they had been programmed to hate me. Even as an escapee, I felt guilty that I might be causing them harm.

The Iranian lawyer, instead, was empowered. "It's not I who . . ." That statement did not lead to my freedom, which had already been achieved, but it stripped away layers of guilt and despair from my heart and even my brain.

We act according to our conscience and principles, not according to evil's attempted manipulations.

Even after recovery, instances reveal themselves from the deep layers of brain, instances where the fear of hurting others (or being hurt yourself, for some) had been used to control you. The life review of the freed entails many times when wrong decisions were made, and a few when right decisions were accomplished. It only takes one or two crucial correct choices to gain freedom, to leave behind the threats and manipulations. With freedom, you have the time to find yourself, long ago lost to perpetrators. You can make the choice to turn your back on your perpetrators fast, but it does take a lifetime to digest all that has happened. You can work through the shock of each tortuous event that occurred in the past, but the post-recovery shock of what your life as a whole has been could stick throughout the rest of your life. Some might be able to shake it off. I have not been able to.

After recovery, you stand as if in shock. This shock will not dissipate by itself. To lose the shock, you have to accept your life. How could anyone accept a life like those that I describe? This is where the flow towards healing can stop. There is no way to accept what happened to you and countless others. No way.

And so we continue. Still grieving and in shock, but we take one step and then another. We have this awful knowledge, but life is calm now and we can help others. We make the best of this life.

The extra danger of character flaws

Wendy Hoffman

The criminal groups test their victims from early childhood on. They want to know what talents and interests they inherited so that they can usurp them for their own purposes. They also want to know what weak spots each personality has in case they need to be punished. Therefore, they ascertain whether a victim will suffer more if he or she is humiliated professionally and in public or whether physical torture would be more effective. Ordinary life schools do not do such thorough investigations.

From my observations, it is survivors' character flaws that keep them attached to the perpetrator group. These blemishes could go unnoticed in ordinary life. Most people have some personality frailty or vulnerability but when unravelling mind control, these deficits can become deadly.

Starved of real recognition (a need of every human), some survivors end up overly hungry for attention, feeling special and important. Perhaps someone held a more special role earlier in life and then lost it. A girl was told to function as a sex goddess and then lost her looks and was demoted. A boy was trained in activities requiring strength but then did not grow very big. A young child showed potential to be a psychic or a witch and these abilities did not develop and crashed. There are many other scenarios that can leave adult survivors longing for some singled out recognition or sense of special importance.

If the cult wants to use the person's abilities in cult life only, the programmers will say, for example,

"Here, with us, you are important."

"We need you."

"You are special."

"Only you can help us."

"Only you have the knowledge and understand."

But if the person is no longer needed or used, he or she is just dropped, humiliated, and closed down, experiencing a hole that flails around to be filled. Only the wrong people will want to fill it.

If you spot this kind of yearning emptiness in yourself, be on guard. Do not fall in love with the handsome leader who tells you you are beautiful. He means you no good. Do not accept that function at a ritual. It is meant to manipulate you. Do not want to be a valued member of a group more than anything. The group will lead you to destruction.

There are survivors who never experienced compassion from others. They were left alone as small children even though their bodies had been tortured. They called out and no one came. No adult. Not even another child. As adults, they remain in that child-state of yearning for comfort from another human being.

We know that in these criminal cults there are programmers who know how to separate victims' brains into slivers and render them unthinking, hypnotised automatons.

There is another group that is not as powerful as programmers but is still used extensively. Members of this group are called "matriarchs." People describe them as being "natural mothers." They have an intuitive sense of how to court people, build them up, and make them dependent. Soon, the comfort-seekers find these matriarchs and stop seeing clearly. They are finally getting the comfort their child selves craved and that blinds them, one hopes temporarily, to the dangerous pit they have fallen into. Apparently supportive partners or spouses can also give comfort while keeping the dependent survivor in a helpless, childish state.

If you are arrested in a small child state of complaining and wanting everyone to comfort you, know that you are courting danger. The wrong people will be happy to rescue you from loneliness and isolation and keep you trapped as a slave who carries out enemies' bidding.

There are adult survivors who, as children, were stripped of any remnant of self-esteem. They believed what their adult and peer torturers told them and think that they have nothing to offer the world. These are the people who will go after the positions of power in these criminal groups and will let sail down the river any whisper their souls or their higher wisdom selves deliver.

If you are a person with such horrendous self-esteem, know that having a position of power in these groups will often seal your fate and render you a doomed victim.

Be aware that you do not feel good about yourself, and protect yourself from enemies who will prey on your lack. Try to spot aspects of yourself that you admire. Remember when you acted with integrity. Yes, there were such times. Push away people who tempt you with destructive forces.

If the cult offers to place you in a high level administrative job in the real world, be cautious. The criminal leaders are not honoring your abilities, though you might want to think so. They are using you as a stooge. They will tell you exactly what to do and how. You might get a large salary but you will remain a puppet with no conscience.

Know your limitations. If you would not be able to achieve such a high position on the basis of your own abilities, do not let empty ambition leave you vulnerable to being used even more and contributing to more of the evil in the world.

Many more character flaws can lead people further into being a puppet of these criminal groups. If you have justifiable rage attacks, the controllers may make you into an assassin. If you tend toward addictions, they may make you into a prostitute or drug pusher or both. If you often become hysterical, they will send a partner who can balance you out and support you but who will not be a friend. The person who helps you cope with histrionic reactions will probably become your handler or programmer. That person may level out your instability but will not want your welfare and will order you to do things to your detriment.

Try to know and accept yourself even though you are mind-controlled and your mind might still be in slivers and pieces. Try to heal your childhood of torture and deprivations so that your enemies cannot place you in an even deeper hole.

Healing from this kind of mind torture is one of the most difficult recoveries. I do not think anyone would disagree about that. Some may even say it is not possible. However, enough people have healed to say definitively that it is possible and happening right now. Minds are becoming integrated.

Satanic mythology *vs.* genuine evil

Alison Miller

A long time ago, people thought bad/unfortunate was the same as bad/evil. So, if someone suffered, it must be a divine punishment for something they had done wrong. Even today, we sometimes confuse these things. People who survive earthquakes, for example, feel especially chosen by God to survive, and thank God for this, without realizing that they are, by implication, thanking God, for killing all those who did not survive. Until recently we called natural disasters "acts of God."

When ancient people realized that what happens to someone is not always his or her fault, they looked for external causes. Many things do have external causes. Not having the science to discover bacteria and viruses and faults in the earth's crust, early people invented mythical beings to account for all the things that go wrong. Ancient religions tend to be filled with deities that are a cross between human beings and animals, some beneficent and some malign. This is probably because, in ancient times, wild animals were one of the greatest threats people faced. A person merged with a powerful beast would have great power. Among other supposedly supernatural beings, people invented a red devil with horns and a tail and a vaguely human or bipedal goat-like body. As time went on, they added more demonic beings, also tending to be red and horned. Recently, in an attempt to explain ritual abuse, some writers (notably David Icke) have added bipedal lizard-like aliens.

Unfortunately, ever since the poet John Milton wrote *Paradise Lost* in 1667, one particular set of mythical beings seem to have won out in the popular imagination. Milton combined three ideas from the Bible to fashion a tale of an entire class of supernatural beings like the Greek or Roman or Egyptian gods, one of whom rebelled against God and took others with him. The ideas he combined were:

1. The adversary or tempter character ("Satan", e.g., in the book of Job, or the story of Jesus in the wilderness) who has the job of testing people's motives to strengthen their character.
2. The notion of "devils" (external forces causing unpleasant effects such as diseases—nowadays we would identify many of them as bacteria or viruses, and others as natural phenomena like the shifting of the earth's crust).
3. A brief reference to Lucifer falling from heaven. Lucifer, the light-bringer, usually referred to the planet Venus, the brightest star in the sky. In its context, the prophet Isaiah was prophesying doom for a foreign king who was oppressing his people, a man who appeared temporarily bright but would be brought down.

Milton, 450 years ago, put these together into an impressive and exciting narrative about an evil being, Lucifer/Satan, who rebelled against God's rule. Many Christians think this story is actually in the Bible; it is not. Satanists, like evangelical Christians, believe it but think the rebel, rather than God, deserves to run the universe. The story is not all that different from similar stories in more ancient mythologies. Ritual abusers who worship Satan or Lucifer often also worship Egyptian or other pagan deities as well. More recent Christians have elaborated on all the demonic entities that supposedly work on behalf of Satan's kingdom.

When I hear the acronym "SRA," standing for satanic ritual abuse, I shudder. People who call what we are dealing with SRA frequently equate mind control abuses, including those engaged in by religious Satan-worshippers, with the involvement of a host of supernatural entities, most of them red and horned and having some kind of a physical body which gives them that appearance. Many such people believe that victims must experience "deliverance" from possession or oppression by such entities.

Various polytheistic religions involve rituals in which people dress up as gods or demons, and go into alternative states in which they are supposedly possessed by the god or demon they represent. Satanism does this also, according to Stella Katz (Chapter Seven of *Healing the Unimaginable*). A man in a devil suit (skin-tight and red with horns and a tail) rapes a toddler in the satanic baptism ceremony, and rapes a nine-year-old painfully (he wears a penis sheath with spikes on it) in the ceremony of marriage to Satan. People wear costumes impersonating demons, and rape a child of about three in order to create demon parts in that child. The child passes out, wakes up costumed as a demon, and is shown a "mirror" on which a picture of demon is painted. It is given a demon name and taught how to behave like a demon.

Most of us do not take literally the various gods and demons of religions other than the ones we are familiar with, Christianity and Judaism. We do not assume that when an ancient Greek or a Mayan dressed in a costume, he actually became, or was possessed by, the entity that costume represented. Yet, somehow, some of us believe this about the demonology we have inherited within Christianity.

Surely our understanding of dissociation can inform us about what has happened within a little child who is raped and tortured into inviting in a "demon" or signing an agreement to serve Satan. The child's brain, in the interest of basic survival, has split off a part that will say or do whatever it is told to say or do. Are we to really believe that some named demon has entered this child, and the only solution is to oust it through "deliverance" or "exorcism?" Surely we are beyond that. Surely we can see that what happened was a dissociative split caused by overwhelming trauma.

Nevertheless, we are faced with the reality that what people do in this kind of religion can only be described as evil. It is impossible to experience or work with victims of mind control abuses, especially ritual abuse, without becoming sickeningly, and frighteningly, aware of the existence of evil. We have to grapple with the reality that the things that happen to mind-controlled and ritually abused people are not just unfortunate examples of "hurt people hurting others." There is deliberate evil intent on the part of perpetrators. Perhaps many or most perpetrators have split minds themselves, so they are unable to feel empathy for their victims. Even the "conscious" ones have hidden child parts, but have lost contact with them.

Forced perpetration is, in my view, the most evil of all the things ritually abusing cults engage in. A little child's hand, in the hand of an adult abuser, is made to stab another creature, perhaps even a person, to death. Older children are given choices between two evils. "Kill this animal or we will kill your baby brother." "Cut this person or we will cut her much more painfully." When they choose the lesser evil, they are told how evil they are for making this choice.

Whenever I hear (or read) someone referring to this kind of abuse as "SRA," I hear the implication that an actual supernatural being who looks like the guy in the red suit is involved. This bothers me immensely. There might well be evil forces beyond our understanding that vie with the good for the heart or soul of each human being. However, literalizing them into physical beings with red skin, horns, and tails takes our focus away from what these abusers may be doing to the humanity of their victims, and what is necessary to restore that humanity.

A client of mine who grew up in a satanic cult family had a near-death experience, in which she died temporarily and had to be revived. When we processed this memory in a therapy session, she went through all the traditional components of the near-death experience, including leaving her body, passing through a tunnel, meeting a being of light, and finally experiencing a review of the choices she had made in her life with regard to whether they were good or evil. In the life review, she reported being shown that some of the evil things she had been made to do by the cult perpetrators were not considered evil choices on her part, as she had not really had a choice between right and wrong. But some smaller decisions in everyday life in which she had chosen to be mean or petty were shown (by the being of light) to be wrong.

Abusers can make very young children believe they are evil or possessed on the basis of the actions those children are forced to commit. But why do we adults believe it? We should know better.

As we learn more about mind control and ritual abuse, we are forced to think through our view of evil, of right and wrong choices, and perhaps of what Christians call "sin." How does a person come to choose evil? How does a person become a perpetrator? Leave aside the forced choices and forced behaviors. What are the choices that count?

Read Wendy's essay on "Character flaws" again. She is talking about temptation, in the traditional sense. The temptation to boost your self-esteem by lording it over others, to deal with your financial insecurity by turning to greed and exploiting others, the temptation to deny your vulnerability by torturing and raping others, the temptation to get love by imprisoning someone and forcing them to "love" you, the temptation to achieve safety by compromising with abusers. Evil enters through temptation, the temptation to violate the Golden Rule, which is "treat others the way you would like them to treat you." A person becomes a perpetrator through a series of such choices.

The cults know this. Forget the trappings of satanism, the costumes, the supposed legions of demons. These are mere window dressing to confuse and deceive and distract children and onlookers. The temptations, even within satanism, are the same old ones that exist anywhere, but with heightened possibilities. Someone who wants to aggrandize himself by making others feel small might, in regular life, become a spouse abuser; in satanism he might become a torturer. In regular life, a smart person who wants to exploit others through greed can become a real estate magnate; a less intelligent person might simply become a loan shark. In satanism, the less smart person can become a university president (with manipulated promotions), the smarter person a master programmer who directs torturers and can rape anyone he wants, including helpless children. In satanism, a person who will sacrifice others in order to avoid personal suffering will become an obedient torturer or a stealer of children. In regular life, he might become a politician who tries to keep vulnerable refugees out of a "safe" country, or a devotee of such a politician. The choices that lead to evil are the same within and outside satanism.

The people who direct the international perpetrator networks know this. They are not deceived by the trappings. As Wendy wrote, they look for the person's individual vulnerability to temptation, and they provide precisely the type of temptation to which each individual is most vulnerable.

As an Illuminati "queen," Wendy was chosen to assume a high position in the international cult network. For this position, she was supposed to be possessed by myriad demons which were simulated through deceptions such as we have previously discussed. But, to her mind, the real evil was not in these supposed demons, it was in the temptation to power and cruelty. Throughout her life she was invited to accept and enjoy the power her position would give her if she would only become a "conscious" perpetrator and identify with the goals of the perpetrator group. Choosing to kill with her own hands was particularly important to the group, and because she steadfastly refused to do so, she was eventually discarded by the group. The boy she grew up with, who was designated to be the "king" to her "queen," lusted after power, and was given significant authority within the group.

Walt Kelly's "Pogo" cartoon for the first Earth Day in 1970 has a caption: "We have seen the enemy, and he is us." There are many people who live regular lives who would become perpetrators if given the opportunity. It is repeated yielding to temptation that destroys the soul. This is a primary objective of satanic groups. The truly demonic takes control of us when we repeatedly yield to what is commonly known as sin—envy, lust for power, control, cruelty, sexual perversion, material possessions, or status. This can happen to anyone, regardless of whether they are exposed to satanism.

SECTION II
LIES

Fifty lies they might have told you: why they told them, how they made you believe them, and what you can do about it

Alison Miller

Child abusers who use mind control, whether they belong to a cult, a military or government group, or an organized criminal group which uses children as sexual slaves, all attempt to brainwash their victims to believe certain lies. "Mind control" refers to deliberately splitting a child's brain circuitry into different parts, training all parts to obey, and indoctrinating and training each part so that he or she will do a specific job assigned by the abusers. The abusers who do this tell the children many lies, for the purpose of controlling the children and preventing them from speaking out about their abuse, even after they grow up, so that the abusers can continue perpetrating these abuses without being caught. In addition, each specific lie has a specific purpose, which benefits the abusers but not the children.

The creation of these false beliefs and trained behaviors is sometimes referred to as "programming." These abusers use trickery (fake stage magic, illusions, and drugs) as well as torture and threats to make children believe the lies. They also deliberately create new parts ("inside people") in each child they abuse. The one or ones who live most of their daily lives and function socially in the outside world often do not know of the beliefs, training, or even the existence of the other parts. This is important for the lies and tricks to be effective. This article summarizes some of the most common lies told by these abusers, the purpose of each lie, and the methods they use to make children believe the lies.

If you are a survivor reading this, I suggest you might want to write down some thoughts you or your parts have that could possibly be lies the perpetrators told you. Then see whether those thoughts are in this list. Or you could ask your inside parts to listen while you read each lie out loud, and note which lies they believe so you can read the explanations of these lies to them.

Lies about the reality of the abuse

1. *Lie*: You got the idea that you were abused from something you read or saw on television, or from someone else's experience, or from your therapist.

The truth: Many people read such stories or watch such programs, but know that these things did not happen to them. All qualified therapists have been trained not to make suggestions that will influence clients' beliefs about what has happened to them.

Why they told this lie: They wanted you to believe that your memories were not real, so that you would not try to find out more about them or tell anyone else about them. They also did not want anyone else to believe you.

How they made you believe it: Survivors of extreme abuse often do not remember much of their past, so it is very easy for people who have power in their lives, such as their parents, to convince them that nothing bad happened to them. Most people want to please their parents.

What to do about it: You might want to avoid reading other people's stories of abuse, or watching television programs about these abuses, whether or not the programs suggest that these things really happen. Then you can be sure that you are not picking up ideas from these sources.

Think seriously about who has made suggestions to you, either that you were abused or that you were not. Can you trust their word? Has anyone pressured you to believe one way or the other? If so, you might want to make it clear to that person that your thoughts are your own and you do not appreciate their suggestions. Possibly the people who deny what you say are part of the perpetrator group.

2. *Lie*: If you get flashbacks of awful abuses, they must be dreams or imagination or signs that you are crazy. Nothing bad really happened to you.

The truth: Flashbacks do not come from imagination, especially if they have body sensations as part of them. Dreams can be related to things you have seen in films or on television, but they might also be related to things that have happened to you. If you have seen screen images which remind your inside parts of their experiences, a dream might combine the story on the screen with actual memories.

Why they told this lie: They wanted you to believe that your memories were not real, so that you would not try to find out more about them or tell anyone else about them.

How they made you believe it: If you had a dream or a memory of the abuse in childhood, they would tell you that it was a dream or that you had an active imagination. It was reassuring to you to believe it was not real. They may have simulated a murder that you attended, and then you saw the person alive the next day. When you told this to your parents, they said you must have dreamed the murder.

What to do about it: Pay attention to dreams and flashbacks; write them down and see what information they give you about your life experiences.

Lies about your abusers' powers and character

3. *Lie*: The abusers know things and do things by real magic.

The truth: The abusers had lots of training in how to deceive children. They used "stage magic," hypnosis, and drugs, as well as torture and threats, to make you believe lies. They did not have any real magic.

Why they told this lie: They wanted you to always be afraid of them and to believe they knew what you were thinking and saying, so that you would not reveal the abuse.

How they made you believe it: You were a child, and children do not always understand adults' tricks. You did not know whether magic was real or not. Stage magicians deceive children for fun; abusers have learned to use this stage magic to deceive children for their evil purposes. For example, a client of mine believed "Satan's eyes" were always watching her. This was a memory of being outside in the dark with the "eyes" she saw being flashlights surrounding her. Another client as a child was put in a room with plastic ears glued to the walls, and talked to someone while a hidden microphone recorded what she said. She was then punished for what she had said, and told that all walls had ears, though some are invisible.

What to do about it: Communicate with your inside parts to find out how each apparently magic trick was done. This article has told you how some of them were done. You may have others. You can find out the tricks by talking inside. The abusers set you up so that each part knows things that other parts do not know. You can find out the truth when you share your knowledge with one another inside your head. You can also look up the comedy duo Penn and Teller, who debunk apparent magic.

4. *Lie*: Everything the abusers told you was true.

The truth: Some things were true, but many things were not true. You can only find out which was which through internal communication.

What to do about it: Think for yourself, now that you are an adult, and critique the information the abusers gave you to see whether or not you now think it could be true. If something is really true, it will resonate as a truth for you. You might find that when something resonates this way, you feel angry or sad, and you might want to avoid thinking about it any further. If this is the case, it will be helpful for you to follow the thread of emotions and thoughts and ask yourself why you are avoiding this. Shed light on it so that you can find the real truth, which is the only way you will be able to heal and to move forward in life. Recognize that if you were deceived, you were a child, so it is not your fault you were deceived. As an adult, you probably still have child parts inside you. Be determined to get at the truth. If one thing the abusers said to you was a lie, then perhaps other things that were said to you were lies or tricks (fabricated events).

5. *Lie*: The perpetrators or the group will always know where you are and what you are saying.

The truth: This was true when you were a child and the abusers had control of you, but it is not true now. They do not have the time or resources to keep track of everyone they have abused, especially people who have relocated to another place, so they train some parts of you to report to them. Older survivors who are far away from their origins might now have no one to report to.

Why they told this lie: They knew they would not have the time or resources to keep track of you at all times once you grew up, but they did not want you to know that and disobey them.

How they made you believe it: (a) They knew where you were in your childhood. When they had you in childhood, they were adults and you were a child. When they abused you, it was in a place that they were in control of. You could only hide in places they knew, so there were not any places you could hide successfully. When they found you, they might say it was by magic, but it was not. Phrases like "Mothers have eyes in the back of their heads" reinforced the belief.

But now that you are an adult, it is unlikely that they can find you easily, especially if you have moved to another town or country. Some of your "inside children" may believe they still live in the places where they were abused; they do not know that your body has grown up and moved to a place where the abusers are not around. Some survivors, though not all, are left alone in adulthood, after the abusers close down their personality systems. They are found only if some part of them tells the abusers they are remembering and talking about the abuse.

(b) Other people. Sometimes, other people, such as your own family members, may have had the job of telling the abusers where you were or what you said when you were a child. They might still have this job. If you are not telling these people things now, the abusers will not know. Often, survivors feel an urge to call a "safe" family member, who is actually not a safe person. Such people also notice and report changes in your energy, hopefulness, body care, friendships, concentration, and learning.

(c) Reporter parts. You probably have one or more inside parts or people who have the job of reporting to your abusers if you ever begin to tell or remember what they did to you. Here's a question to think about: Why would the abusers need parts of you to report to them where you are or what you have said, if they already know? The answer is that they would not. They gave parts the job of reporting because they knew that when you are an adult they would not be able to keep track of what you do or say. If there is some part of you who feels he or she just *has* to tell your mother, brother, uncle or somebody from your childhood what you are saying or what you do in therapy, be suspicious. Make sure that part does not act on this impulse.

(d) Hidden microphones. Reporter parts are trained through tricks usually involving microphones. When you were a child, they might have put you in a room where they had hidden a microphone. They would listen to whatever you said when you thought they were not listening, and then they came in and punished you for what you said. They might have told you that they knew by magic, or that some small animal or bird or insect told them, or that they watched from the shadows, or that there was something like a microphone or transmitter which they put in your body which let them know your location, or that the walls had ears. All these were lies. The reporter parts were the ones punished, and they were told they always had to tell what they had said or where they were before they got punished for not telling. The truth is that the rooms you are in now do not have hidden microphones so no one outside these rooms can hear what you say.

What to do about it: Look for your reporter parts and explain to them why they should not report anything you have told anyone about what happened to you. If they report regularly, have them just say that nothing has been done or said against the rules of the group who abused you. The truth now is that if your reporter parts do not tell the abusers things, the abusers will not know. So, it is very important that the reporters stop reporting the truth to the abusers. If they are supposed to call at regular times, they can just talk about unimportant things or even tell lies. The abusers lied to you, so why should you not lie to them? See Lie #6 about lying to abusers. If the reporter parts do not believe they are safe and refuse to cooperate, do not disclose abuses until you and your therapist have worked with these parts sufficiently to get their cooperation. They might agree to be put to sleep when you talk to your therapist about what happened to you, or to have their memories wiped by other parts who know how to do it, so that they will not have to report about disclosures. Or you can have them report to "inside copies" of the abusers.

6. *Lie*: Your abusers always know if you are lying, so you must always tell the truth to them or you will be punished.

The truth: There has been a lot of research into whether or not people can tell when other people are lying, and they cannot. Your abusers cannot tell if you lie to them.

How they made you believe it: When you were a child, your family and/or abusers knew a lot about your life. They may have set you up to lie to them about something they already knew, then punished you for lying.

What to do about it: Realize that although in most situations telling the truth is the right thing to do, there are some situations (when someone's life or health, including your own, is at stake), it may be right to lie, especially to people who cannot be trusted. If you decide to lie to your abusers, practice that lie so you can do it effectively.

7. *Lie*: You can trust the people who abused you, your "family," but you cannot trust anyone else.

The truth: There are many people who are trustworthy and will not betray you or let you down. You cannot trust people who are part of a group that abuses children. Your abusers are the very people you can never trust, whether or not they are your biological family. They are the people who abused you, and who made you watch or take part in abuses of helpless children, adults, and animals. How could you possibly trust people who have behaved like this, regardless of how "nice" or "normal" they might seem at other times? You can rely on the fact that they will hurt you and lie about it!

How they made you believe it: They had someone whom you believed was not one of them hurt you or betray your trust. That person was actually one of them. They may have had a family member or a cult member rescue you. They arranged your personality system so that the parts who were rescued do not know the abuse which the other parts experienced by family or group members, including the same people who rescued you.

Also, when you were very young, they might have set up some kind of a trick situation, where you had to choose between people whom you believed were outsiders to the perpetrator group or family, and members of that group or family. If you chose to go to the outsiders, they abused you. If you chose to go to the group members, they were nice to you and rewarded you. The trick was that the people who were supposedly "outsiders" were not really outsiders; they were just group members you had not met before. And the group members who were nice to you were not always nice in this way but some part in you created just for this situation did not know that.

What to do about it: When all your internal parts share information with one another, you can discover the lie in this kind of training. Some part who is older than the one trained here can share what he or she knows about what else those "outsiders" and those "nice people" did at other times.

Do not trust anyone who has abused you at any time. Many abusers in these perpetrator groups are dissociative, and their "nice" parts may not even know what their abusive parts do.

With true outsiders, take your time to evaluate whether or not you can trust them. Share information internally so that those parts of you who make the decisions have all the necessary information to know whether people are trustworthy. Many people can be trusted with some information but not with everything you have to tell.

8. *Lie*: The group can kill you or take you away at any time and no one can stop it from happening.

The truth: It is very risky for an abuser group to kill someone or permanently kidnap them. If that person is known in the world, there will be an investigation, and abuser groups do not want that to happen. The victims they kill are usually street people or unregistered children (whom no outsiders know exist), not people with real-world identities. Groups can temporarily kidnap survivors to re-abuse them, but they let them go. In the past they kidnapped children and sometimes killed adults with known identities, but it is now almost always too risky for them to do this, particularly if the person has disclosed abusers' identities to an outsider like a safe therapist or doctor.

How they made you believe it: You probably saw the abusers appear to kill someone, or even kidnap a child, back in the days when parents did not watch their children as closely as they do now.

What to do about it: Know that you are very probably safe from being killed or permanently abducted, but if an abuser group actually knows where you are, take precautions so that they will not take you somewhere and re-abuse you.

Survivors who come from very high-ranking cult families, who are being used in important jobs for the perpetrator group, or who have knowledge of publicly known crimes, are likely to be tracked more thoroughly than rank-and-file survivors. Unfortunately, modern technology makes it easier to discover someone's address, or follow them via tracking their cellphone. So if you are one of those survivors who is important to the perpetrator group, you may have to be extra careful not to make yourself vulnerable to abduction. You also have to remember that some cult people are experts in disguises and know how to con people and present a likeable front, and may try to befriend you. For example, if they hear that you are ill, they might move in to "help" you, but will actually torture you.

Lies about obedience and disobedience

9. *Lie*: You are "good" if you obey the abusers, and "bad" if you do not.

The truth: You know deep inside what is good and bad. It is bad to hurt people or animals. The abusers use "good" to mean obedient and "bad" to mean disobedient. But there is a higher form of goodness, based on the Golden Rule—"treat other people the way you would like them to treat you." If obeying someone means violating the Golden Rule, it is not really good at all. Somewhere deep down inside you, you know this. You did not want to obey many times because you knew what they were doing was wrong. Most of the time what the abusers told you to do was bad, even though they told you it was good.

Why they told this lie: To confuse you and to make you disobey your own conscience. Children believe what adults say, and trust the adults to know better than they do.

How they made you believe it: They said it a lot. They talked all the time, as many parents do, about being "good" in terms of obedience. If you refused to do something you knew would hurt yourself or someone else, they said you were bad. They punished you for trying to escape, for talking to outsiders, for acts of kindness. They punished you for being disobedient, and they sometimes rewarded you for being obedient.

What to do about it: You still have your conscience, and underneath all the training the abusers gave to parts of you, you still know that it is right to care for yourself and other people and wrong to hurt yourself or others. Know that the guilty and fearful feelings you get when you disobey the abusers is just left over from all the punishment and lies they told you. Trust in your own inner knowledge of what is good and bad. If you are in doubt, ask someone you trust who is not one of the abusers. Try to get back to the higher morality of the Golden Rule, and base your behavior on trying to treat others and yourself with kindness and compassion rather than having to obey anyone who would make you do harm.

10. *Lie*: You have to remain loyal and obedient to the people who abused you, because you made vows or promises to them. If you do not, you are a traitor and deserve punishment.

The truth: Vows or promises made by children are not legally valid. Children who are forced to make vows or promises under duress, including "marriage" vows, are not legally bound to keep those promises. Even if you signed an agreement or contract consciously as an adult, it is not valid if it was coerced or signed by one part of you without the knowledge of the main "real world" person.

Why they told you this lie: They used your desire to be a loyal person who keeps your word, as well as your fear of death and pain, to make you keep their crimes a secret.

How they made you believe it: Many children abused by organized perpetrator groups were forced to watch a supposed "traitor" being tortured, raped, and/or apparently murdered, and sometimes forced to hold the knife or other instrument that was used. Some of these crimes are simulated, but others are real, and the children forced to be there believe they are real.

Under this kind of duress, a child splits off parts that are desperate to be loyal. When these parts do what is required of them, including making vows, they are rewarded by the abusers.

What to do about it: Vows made by a child under duress are not legally valid, so you do not have to do anything other than recognize this.

Some survivors like to make formal statements which deliberately contradict the vows they were forced to make, for example, "divorcing Satan" if they were "married" to him.

11. *Lie*: If you disobey your abusers, someone you love, or your pet, or another vulnerable child will be punished or will die.

The truth: When you were a child, they could punish someone else to make you obey their instructions. If you are still in contact with the perpetrators now, and they want to continue to use you, they are able to punish someone else (though they are unlikely to actually kill that person). But they will only do it when you are present to watch or take part. If you are no longer in physical contact with them, no one will be harmed because you disobey their instructions. They will continue harming other children, but you have no control over that, only over how you yourself can become and stay safe. Children and adult survivors do not need abusers, even if they are mothers, fathers, brothers, sisters, grandparents, sons, daughters, best friends, spouses, or lovers.

How they made you believe it: When you disobeyed as a child, they punished a younger child, perhaps your little brother or sister, for your disobedience. Or they harmed or killed a child or an animal and told you it was because of your disobeying them. They might even have made you harm someone, telling you that if you did not do it they would harm you as well as that person, or they would hurt that person worse than you would. They did this when you were a child under their control in order to make you do things you would not otherwise agree to do. They used your own love and compassion against you.

What to do about it: Refuse to believe this lie, and keep yourself physically safe and away from any of the abusers. Do not return to them and give them the opportunity to harm you or someone else in your presence. If you are unable to keep physically away from the abusers, consider relocating to another part of the country or the world, but only do this when no part of you is reporting your location to the abusers.

12. *Lie*: Your internal leaders must always make the other parts obey, and punish them if they disobey, or the abusers will find these inner people and punish them severely.

The truth: Your abusers probably did put some inner "people" in charge of the others, and instruct them to keep all parts of you obeying the abusers' instructions through threats and punishments. However, if you have physically moved away from your abusers, and they are no longer able to physically capture and punish you, your internal leaders no longer have to perform internal punishments and give warnings. The abusers will not punish these leaders if they stop doing their jobs, because they can only punish any parts of you if they have your body to punish.

Why they told this lie: They wanted to continue to have control of you when you were far away from them. They knew that you would grow up and move away, so they gave those parts the job of making everyone inside you continue to obey them.

How they made you believe it: It was actually true when you were a child and under the control of the abusers. Those parts were put in charge and punished if any parts under their authority disobeyed. But the abusers can only do this if they have your body to punish.

What to do about it: Make sure that all parts, especially those who were put in charge, know what year it is, how old your body is, where you live, and how far away you are from your abusers. Many parts can be "stuck in the past" and still think it is 1968 or 1987 or some other year when you were still physically a child and the abusers were in charge of you. The parts who were put in charge need to be fully informed about the situation, and if they realize they are no longer in danger, then they can stop punishing the others and learn to work together with all parts for your safety and healing.

13. *Lie*: If you do as you are told, you will rise to be the highest member of the coven.

The truth: Ritual abusers say this to every child they abuse. Every ritually abused child has within him or her parts such as the high priest or priestess, the bride of Satan, and possibly the programmers. These lies are told to these parts to keep them in line. The persons to lead the next generation of the group are usually chosen at birth, and no one else can rise to those positions.

How they made you believe it: By creating these parts and telling them these lies. There are many reasons parts of you would want to believe this—it would give them some importance, safety, and a sense of purpose and belonging.

What to do about it: Just realize you were lied to.

Lies about keeping in contact with your abusers

14. *Lie*: If you go to the abusers, you will not be punished, and if you obey and go back, you will get a special treat.

The truth: If you have been disloyal in any way, such as going to see a safe therapist or telling anyone anything about the abuse, you will be punished when you return to the abusers. The "special treat" could be a chance to harm or kill some creature, with a cheap ring and a fake "promotion" given to you afterward. Or it might be a chance to be hurt. You may be rewarded with sex or given drugs in an attempt to get you addicted.

If you do not go to them, they will not be able to hurt you or to make you hurt any other creature.

How they made you believe it: There might have been an event in your childhood where you were rewarded for going to them.

What to do about it: Do not go to them! Try to educate those parts who go to them about what actually happens when you get there, so they will not want to go there anymore.

15. *Lie*: If you do not return to the abusers on birthdays and other special dates, they will hurt someone else.

The truth: They will only do this if you are there to watch or to be forced to take part in hurting the other person.

How they made you believe it: On one or more occasions in childhood you were late or did not show up for one of their events, when they were still in control of you. As a punishment, they hurt someone else while you watched, or made you hurt someone.

What to do about it: Make sure that you do not go back to the abusers. They might still hurt other people, of course, but not because of you. You might want to change the date on which you celebrate your birthday, or just pretend you do not have a birthday at all.

16. *Lie*: If you do not return to the abusers on birthdays and other special dates, they will hunt you down and punish you.

The truth: This might be true if you still live in the vicinity of your abusers. It is not true if you live far away from them. They cannot just leave their lives and travel across the continent or the world to find you, and force you to travel back with them.

How they made you believe it: They played games when you were a child, during which you had to hide and they inevitably found you. They did hunt you down and punish you when you were a child if you tried to be absent from one of their events.

What to do about it: Assess carefully whether you are far enough away from the abusers. You might need to make careful plans to move away from them if they are still able to abduct you easily. If you plan to move away, make sure that no inside "reporter" reports your plans and your new location to the abusers.

17. *Lie*: If you do not tell the abusers what you have told outsiders about them, the abusers will know you have told outsiders, and will hunt you down and punish you.

The truth: If you do not report to the abusers, they will know nothing about what you have or have not told others (as long as those others were not people sent by the abuser group.)

Why they told this lie: To protect themselves from being punished for their crimes; to stop any possible exposure of their crimes as quickly as possible.

How they made you believe it: See Lie #3 under "Lies about abusers' powers", above. They triggered you to tell someone, and listened with a hidden microphone, when you were a child. Or the person you told was actually one of them. There are no hidden microphones now, the walls do not have ears, there is no all-seeing eye that will see you, and no creatures will report to the abusers if you do not report to them. Those were all lies they told to convince you that they know whatever you say. There are still people who seem safe but are actually part of the group, however.

What to do about it: Make sure that the reporter parts do not report to abusers. If you have to talk to a family member who is part of the abusive group, make sure that reporter parts are ready to lie or do not know anything you have told an outsider.

18. *Lie*: You always have to answer the phone, or something bad will happen.

The truth: Your phone is under your control. Nothing will happen if you do not answer it.

Why they told this lie: They wanted you to always be accessible to them, to report about your life and any disclosures you have made, and to be told where and when to go back to them.

How they made you believe it: They set up a scenario when you were a child where you were punished by them or by someone impersonating "Satan" when you did not answer the phone.

What to do about it: Turn your phone to voicemail, get Call Display, and then you can decide whether or not to answer calls or to listen to messages.

19. *Lie*: Even on the phone, inside parts of you have to come out if they are asked for.

The truth: Your abusers do not actually know which part of you they are talking to.

Why they told this lie: They wanted to have complete control of you, and part of that control is getting out the parts who are too fearful to disobey them.

How they made you believe it: They punished you until the part they wanted would come out, so all the parts learned to come out when called out.

What to do about it: Try to avoid talking with any abusers who might call out parts. But if you do find yourself talking to them, remember that they do not know which part they are talking to, and keep a strong part out who will not obey them or is capable of lying to them when they ask questions which could get you into trouble.

20. *Lie*: You always have to answer the door and open it, even if you do not want to see the person who comes to the door.

The truth: You are an adult and your life is your own. If you have a good sturdy lock on your door, you do not have to open it to anyone you do not want to see, and they will not break the door down now.

Why they told this lie: They wanted to be able to get hold of you and re-abuse you after you moved away from them.

How they made you believe it: They might have broken down a door and punished you as a child if you locked a door against them.

What to do about it: Keep a strong lock on your door and make sure that no part of you comes out to unlock and open the door if your abusers come to the door.

Lies about what will happen if you tell

21. *Lie*: It is not safe to tell anyone what happened to you. If you tell a therapist or a doctor they will disbelieve you, say you are crazy, and lock you up in a mental institution where you will be drugged, restrained, and possibly abused. They might actually abuse you themselves.

The truth: A therapist or doctor who is not part of the perpetrator group will not personally abuse you if you tell them what happened. There is a chance that they will think you are mentally ill, lock you up in a mental hospital, and/or put you on drugs to treat your "illness." However, it is actually difficult to get admitted to a psychiatric facility these days, and even if you were admitted, you would likely be out in a few days. There is also a chance that they will believe you and give you the help that you need. It depends on how well educated they are about abuse and trauma. You will not be abused in hospital unless the group who abused you has access to that hospital. Some hospitals are safe and supportive for survivors; some are not.

Why they told this lie: They do not want their secrets discovered because their acts were crimes, and they could be tried and imprisoned for what they did to you.

How they made you believe it: When you were a child or a teenager you might have been taken to a "therapist" or a "doctor" who was actually one of the abuser group. They might have abused you in their office. They might have put you in a place you believed to be a mental institution and given you strong drugs which made you feel crazy, and you might have been abused there. This was a trick to make you think that therapists and doctors who are not part of the abuser group cannot be trusted.

(a) Many children who are being abused on an ongoing basis are taught not to go to doctors about their injuries or illnesses. Doctors attached to the abusive group treat them and often abuse them.

Parents who permit their children to be abused, or who abuse them, do not want any doctor who is not part of the perpetrator group to discover injuries, because they could then get in trouble with the law, and their children could be taken from them and put into safe foster homes. If a child is abused so badly that he or she has to be hospitalized, the parents lie to the doctors and social workers, and the child is too frightened to talk because he or she will be returned to the family.

(b) In some cases, the group may have used real doctors or therapists who were members of their group. But this does not mean that all such people belong to these groups. Most doctors and most therapists are sincere, good people who want to help. However, many of them are completely unaware that there are groups who torture and brainwash children, and some might find it difficult to believe and might think you are deluded.

What to do about it: Therapists can be enormously helpful to survivors of extreme and organized child abuse. However, not all therapists understand dissociation and people who have other "parts" or "people" inside. If possible, the therapist you choose to talk to will be recommended by someone you trust (not a family member or another unhealed survivor). Ideally, he or she should have experience both with people with different parts inside and with survivors of the kind of abuse you experienced.

However, do not tell the therapist a lot of information about the abuses you suffered until you know that your therapist is not part of the abuser group, and no inside part of you is reporting your disclosures to the abusers. If the reporters do not report, the abusers do not know you are talking to an outsider. If the reporters do report to the abusers, the group will do something to make you stop talking.

Once you are sure that no part of you is reporting your disclosures to the abusers, go ahead and talk to your therapist. You need to talk about what happened to you in order to recover from it. Your abusers will not know, and you will be safe with the therapist, as long as the therapist is not part of the abuser group.

If you have an illness or injury, it is wise to go to a medical professional to have it assessed and treated. However, do not go to the one you had in childhood unless you are 100% sure that person is safe. Most doctors are not involved with perpetrator groups. A doctor can also document any visible injuries from your abuse.

22. *Lie*: It is not safe to tell the police what happened to you. They will lock you up in prison because you are a murderer or a rapist. You will be abused when you are locked up.

The truth: A court will never jail someone for crimes in which they were forced to participate as a child. Children are not responsible for these crimes; the adults who made them take part are responsible.

Why they told this lie: They do not want their secrets discovered because their acts were crimes, and the adults could be tried and imprisoned for what they did to you.

How they made you believe it: When you were a child you may have been introduced to an abuser you did not know dressed in a police uniform, and triggered to tell this person something that the abusive group did to you. You might have been triggered to remember and tell about a crime in which you were forced to participate. The "police officer" (who was actually one of the abuser group) then abused you, said you were a murderer or a rapist, and locked you up in a place you believed to be a prison, where he or other "officers" or "inmates" abused you.

What to do about it: It is probably unwise to talk to law enforcement about what happened to you until and unless you have your memories completely clear and you are far away from where the abuse happened. The police will not lock you up or call you a criminal or abuse you themselves. However, police have to talk to the alleged abusers, who will then know you are talking about what they did and could decide to come and punish you. You might need to report your abuses in order to get funding for therapy from a crime victims' assistance fund, and other state or county benefits. This is a safe thing to do as long as you are far away from your abusers. If you do talk to the police, it is wise to have a good therapist with you or at least seeing you regularly when you do this.

23. *Lie*: There is a bomb inside you. If you talk about the abuse, the bomb will go off and kill you and anyone near you.

The truth: There is no bomb inside you.

Why they told this lie: They did not want the dirty secrets of their abuse revealed.

How they made you believe it: They did a fake operation, putting you to sleep in a place that appeared to be a hospital and having you wake up with a bandage. They might have showed you an X-ray of the bomb inside someone. That X-ray was of someone else's body, not yours. They probably used the same X-ray for all the children.

What to do about it: Help those inner people or parts involved in this memory to discover how the trick was done. Have them share with one another all parts of the memory.

24. *Lie*: There is a creature inside you. If you talk about the abuse, the creature will eat you up from inside.

The truth: There is no creature inside you.

Why they told this lie: They did not want the dirty secrets of their abuse revealed.

How they made you believe it: They might actually have put a real creature in a body cavity, then removed it when you were unconscious or had a different part of you out in the body.

What to do about it: Help those inner people or parts involved in this memory to discover how the trick was done. Have them share with one another all parts of the memory.

25. *Lie*: People you tell about the abuse and their families will be hurt or killed.

The truth: Organized abusers do not kill people who have identities in the real world; it is too risky because there would be an investigation.

How they made you believe it: When you were a child, they might have given you someone to talk to about the abuse, and then killed or pretended to kill that person.

What to do about it: Keep on talking to people you know you can trust, especially your therapist. The more you tell, the more careful the group will be not to get discovered. But get all your inside parts to agree to this so that some of them do not punish you for telling outsiders. It may be difficult to get them to agree, but while you wait for consensus, those parts whom the abusers put in charge can give new orders that everyone must obey—that you should talk and not keep the cult's evil secret.

Lies about life and death and reality

26. *Lie*: Your life will always be so unbearable that it is better to die.

The truth: The feeling that your life is unbearable is a feeling from a memory when your abusers made you feel this way through a combination of drugs and torture and verbal abuse. There may be parts inside you whose job is to give you flashbacks and body memories, especially memories of times when you were made to harm someone. If you have escaped from the abusers, your life can become much happier when these parts stop doing the jobs the abusers assigned them.

Why they told this lie: They wanted you to be dead rather than telling the world about the horrible things they were doing.

How they made you believe it: They put you, as a child, in an unbearable situation, in which you were not only abused but also told repeatedly that you were worthless, a waste of space, and ought to be dead. They then instructed some parts to make you feel the feelings from this awful situation if you began to remember or talk about the abuse.

What to do about it: Find the parts who are making you have these feelings, and help them know that you are now safe and they no longer have to force you to feel this way; nothing will happen to them if they stop doing this.

27. *Lie*: If you (a particular inside person) kill the body, you will not die.

The truth: If the only body you have in this real world is killed, all parts of you will die. Even if you have a separate body from the others in your inside world, you share the same body with them in the real world outside.

How they made you believe it: They split off a part who could not feel anything in the body, probably because of anesthetic drugs. They told that part that he or she was not one of you, and did not belong to the body. They promised that part a great reward if he or she killed the body. They might have given that part a taste of the reward—strong "happy" drugs or enjoyable sex, or food after being starved. This is no different from the training of the assassins and suicide bombers trained in the Middle East with hashish to believe that they will go to paradise to enjoy sexual pleasures.

What to do about it: Again, do not believe the lies. You can test to see whether any inside being is part of the body this way: Mark something on your hand. Then ask that being to come out and see whether or not what you have marked is on its hand.

28. *Lie*: It is honorable to die for the cause of the abusers.

The truth: There is no honor in dying for the beliefs of someone who forced you to obey them when you were a child, without knowing whether those beliefs are right. The honorable thing is to find out whether those beliefs are really true and are worth giving your life for.

How they made you believe it: They pounded this idea into your head, telling you not to think, just to obey. They made you repeat their beliefs and your vows of loyalty and your promise to die for the cause. They might have told you that you are a soldier in a great army.

What to do about it: Think for yourself. You have a choice. Decide what all parts of you together believe. Do not give away your most precious possession, your life, for things you were brainwashed to believe.

29. *Lie*: Dead people can come back to life if they have special powers.

The truth: No one has the power to become alive again once they are dead, although doctors can restart the heart of someone who dies in hospital if they do it right away.

How they made you believe it: You saw someone important killed, but it was actually a trick. Then, when you saw that person alive again they told you it was because he had special powers.

What to do about it: You do not have to believe what adults told you when you were little. Ask your parts if any of them know what trick was used to make you think a person was actually killed when that person was alive later. For example, a bag of blood could be placed on top of the person and stabbed.

30. *Lie*: Eating someone's flesh and drinking human blood makes you wise and powerful.

The truth: Some occult religious groups and cannibalistic tribes believe this. If this were the case, the people who abused you would really be wise as well as powerful in the real world. Usually they are not.

How they made you believe it: You were a child when they told you this, and you believed what adults say.

What to do about it: You are now old enough to think for yourself and decide the beliefs that make sense to you, not to blindly follow what you were told.

31. *Lie*: Spiders, worms, snakes, or insects will eat you alive or bite or sting you to death.

The truth: Most of these creatures are just harmless creatures and do not eat people.

How they made you believe it: When you were very little, they put you in among these creatures and told you that if you moved or made a sound these creatures would bite you, sting you, or eat you up. You believed what adults told you.

What to do about it: Read or watch nature shows about the creatures you are afraid of so that you can learn the truth about them.

32. *Lie*: Everyone you know is linked to the abuser group and knows your every move, and will report back to your abusers.

The truth: Most people do not even know about the kind of abuse you experienced, and would be shocked to hear about it. However, some well-meaning people might not believe that people can do such evil things, and might talk to your family members, believing that you need help for such crazy thoughts. This is particularly true for children and teens. Also, especially if you are of high value to the abuser group, they may have encouraged you to move into a neighbourhood where many people were part of the group, and they may have selected friends for you who were part of the group.

How they made you believe it: They introduced you to people you thought were not part of the group, and they did turn out to be group members, who were sent to you by the group.

What to do about it: Take your time in getting to know people and do not blurt out your experiences to everyone. See whether they can be trusted with smaller disclosures, and if they can, then you can tell them more. However, if you are of high value to the cult and are being pursued in adulthood, it is wise not to speak about the organized abuse at all unless you are certain the person you are speaking to is not part of the group. Be cautious about people who rush in to befriend you if you move to a new location. Watch people for inconsistencies in behaviors or opinions, such as saying "we" instead of "I," which would show they might be multiple. Notice whether they forget things they have previously said. If you know one person in a group belongs to a criminal cult, be suspicious of the other people in this person's group. Satanists often cluster together. Make up your mind that being alone is not the worst thing.

Lies about who you are

33. *Lie*: If you have been made to harm some person or animal, you are evil and a perpetrator, rather than a victim.

The truth: When you were made to do this, you were in an impossible situation, and you were not there of your own free will. You would not blame the knife for what a person made it do. You were in the same situation as the knife, being used as a tool or a weapon rather than choosing to do evil, even though you might have been used by adults to accomplish evil things.

How they made you believe it: They put you in a situation where a helpless person or animal was being hurt or even killed, and they forced you to take part in this, either by physically holding you in position and moving your arm, or by threats of death to you and/or those you loved if you did not comply with their orders. If you refused, they hurt you or the other victim until you split off a part who would do what they wanted. They then told you that you were evil and "special" like them, that you belonged to them, no one else would ever want you, and that if you ever told anyone about what happened, you would be arrested and charged for the crime.

What to do about it: Although you may feel sorrow and remorse about what happened, do not believe the lie that you were responsible for it. You endured spiritual abuse by being made a part of these crimes. Get acquainted with the parts of yourself who refused to do these things, so that you can see that you as a whole person would never choose this evil. Those parts were probably discarded by the perpetrator group, and they will add strength to you when you find them.

34. *Lie*: Your abusers live inside you.

The truth: Everyone who lives inside you is a part of you and is not anyone else.

Why they told this lie: They wanted you to believe they were present when you grew up and they were actually far away from you.

How they made you believe it: Organized abusers like to create parts who are supposed to be internal copies of themselves. Those parts are supposed to speak to the others in their voice, do whatever they do, and bring back memories of the abuses they have done to the other parts, particularly if the other parts disobey and try to get well.

What to do about it: If you hear the abusers' voices, those are either the voices of the internal parts who are supposed to "be" the abusers, or they are memories of the abusers replayed by parts whose job is to make you believe the abusers are inside you. You may notice that the voices always say the same thing in the same way: that is because they are "playbacks" of memories. There are other parts inside who make you hear these voices. Speak to the parts who make you hear those voices, tell them they are also hurt children like you, and they do not have to be the abusers or obey them any longer. Offer them new names and new things to do, jobs which are more interesting than impersonating abusers who cannot hurt you now. For example, parts who play tapes of scary voices can play relaxing music inside.

35. *Lie*: God hates you because of the evil you have done—or, God approves what this group does and hates you because you do not obey your orders.

The truth: Those who believe in God, the good force in the universe, believe that He does not hate people; God only hates evil itself. Many survivors, or parts of survivors, never wanted to participate in evil, but were given forced "lesser of two evils" choices. God would never reject them, and would feel only compassion for them. Others may have been tempted by rewards, or traded someone else's safety for their own. Those who believe in a good God would say that when someone is truly sorry for having participated in evil, God willingly forgives them.

Why they told this lie: They wanted you to feel you had been rejected by God so that you would only go to them and their deities (like Satan or Lucifer) for acceptance.

How they made you believe it: Some human man impersonated God or Jesus when you were a child, and told you he hated you and wanted nothing to do with you because you were evil. He might have abused you as well.

What to do about it: Recognize that this was a trick. Try to find your own spirituality by connecting to the powerful and loving force of good in the universe, who will accept you, and forgive you if you are in need of forgiveness.

36. *Lie*: If you love or get attached to people or animals, something bad will happen to them.

The truth: Nothing will happen to any person you love because you love them, either through you, by the perpetrator group, or by magic. However, the perpetrators sometimes hurt pets.

How they made you believe it: They either harmed or forced you to harm, maybe even kill, someone you loved when you were a small child. They may have held your hands around the knife that the executioner was using. Then they told you repeatedly that you are evil and that the evil in you would harm anyone you got close to. They pretended this was happening, and may have simulated harm to someone who was near you. They may have told you to kill someone psychically, then had someone fall down to make you believe you had killed that person. They may have told you that they will kill anyone you tell about what they did.

What to do about it: Do not believe the lies. Seek out safe friends. Form an attachment to your therapist if he or she is good; this attachment to a good person will help you heal from the evil you were exposed to.

37. *Lie*: You have animals, demons, monsters, aliens, or other people's spirits inside you.

The truth: Everyone inside you is a part of you, no matter how they behave or what they look like in your inner world.

Why they told this lie: They wanted to keep most parts of you afraid to disobey, so they made some parts look and sound frightening to the others, and told them to punish or frighten the other parts so they would not disobey the abusers' instructions.

How they made you believe it: When you were a young child, they used trickery to make you believe these things. They drugged you, dressed you up in a costume, and told you that you were a demon, an animal, a monster, or an alien. They may have shown you a "mirror" which was really just a picture of some creature pasted on top of the mirror, not a real mirror. They did things to your body and told you they were putting their spirit or their seed in you, so they would be inside you. These experiences were so frightening that you split off parts who believed the lies, and these parts were given instructions to growl or to say frightening things.

What to do about it: Recognize that all parts of you who appear to be something else are really just child parts, who were hurt and told lies. Help them know that you are safe now, so they can take off their costumes, stop doing the jobs they were given, and be children again.

38. *Lie*: You are the child of the devil and belong only to the abusers who worship him.

The truth: If you were born in a garage, that does not make you a car. And being born into a coven family does not make you their property. You are a free human being and can choose who you will belong to and how you behave.

How they made you believe it: Some of your parts have no memories except the ones of being in rituals or other abusive scenarios. So they believed what they were told about who they were.

What to do about it: Share the other kinds of memories, such as school and friendships, with them, and help them understand that you are all parts of one child who was horribly abused.

39. *Lie*: You are going to hell, and will be there for eternity with Satan or Lucifer, and your only choice is whether you will be hurt there or hurt others.

The truth: No one in this life knows exactly what happens after we die. Nothing you have done in this life, especially if you were forced to do it, has earned you an eternity in hell.

How they made you believe it: They may have simulated "hell" with fire and dry ice for smoke, and people in devil costumes, in a place here on earth. They hurt you and they may have given some of your parts the choice of doing the hurting rather than being hurt. They might have made a part of you believe she was Satan's or Lucifer's bride through a sexual act by a person impersonating him, and they may have made a part believe he or she was Satan's or Lucifer's child because it was split off by a rape by someone in a costume, putting in his "seed" (sperm). (This can be done to boys as well as girls.)

What to do about it: Recognize that these were all tricks done when you were a child, that "hell" was not really the afterlife but a place on earth, and that your abusers have no control over what happens after you die. Tell the parts who were forced to hurt others that they were tricked, and they do not have to take the abusers' side to avoid being harmed after death. Develop your own understanding of what happens after death rather than taking anyone's word for it.

Recognize that being raped by someone in a devil or Beast costume does not make you either his bride or his child; it makes you his victim. Disown your "husband" or "father" or false "god."

40. *Lie*: You are going to heaven, where you will have to spend eternity with God or Jesus telling you that you are bad, and punishing you.

The truth: No one in this life knows exactly what happens after we die. It is up to you whether or not you believe in God or Jesus. Know, however, that those sincere souls who believe in God or in Jesus see him as being good, kind, and forgiving, not as punishing through torture.

How they made you believe it: Different survivors' experiences differ here. You may have been sexually abused and/or rejected by a priest, or told by a priest or minister that God rejected you or that you needed to have sex with him in order for God to forgive you. Abusers might have simulated "heaven" with someone in a costume pretending to be God or Jesus. At Christmas, you might have been forced to kill what you believed was the baby Jesus. At Easter you might have been forced to participate in nailing someone to a cross. Then "God" or "Jesus" rejected you, verbally and possibly physically abused you, and may even have raped you.

What to do about it: Realize that the people who hurt you were not God or Jesus, but human beings from the abuser group. Realize that if you had to hurt or kill anyone, it was not your free choice, and that person can forgive you, and that person was not really God or Jesus. That person might or might not have really died, but you were not responsible for it.

Align yourself with the good spiritual force that is within all humanity and all of nature, and reject the evil that the abusers forced upon you. Ask forgiveness from anyone you have hurt, in your imagination if not in person.

41. *Lie*: You have special powers that can be used at any time to destroy people's lives.

The truth: You have no special powers. Even if you have some psychic ability, many people (and animals) have that and scientific studies show that it is generally not very reliable.

How they made you believe it: They may have staged a situation in which you believed you killed or harmed someone just by being with them or by using the "power" they trained you in. It was all a trick.

What to do about it: Do not be tempted by the illusion of special powers. Instead, learn how to cooperate with all your parts internally so that you can become a peaceful, healthy human being with all parts working together for recovery.

42. *Lie*: People you know and like or love will always leave you and end up hating you.

The truth: People like those who treat them kindly, and do not like those who mistreat them. However, infiltrators from the perpetrator group usually start by appearing unusually helpful and kind.

How they made you believe it: They told you repeatedly that people would abandon you. They might have allowed you to become friends with someone who then turned on you. This was a setup; the other person was obeying their orders.

What to do about it: Choose your own friends from among the people who treat you with kindness, after checking with all your insiders about whether those people are consistently kind and honest. Treat them the way you would like them to treat you, and they will not leave you or hate you.

43. *Lie*: Your brain or your heart has been replaced by that of another person or creature.

The truth: Every part of your body is the original part you were born with.

Why they told this lie: They wanted complete control over you, and they wanted you to believe that your body belonged to them rather than to you.

How they made you believe it: When you were a young child, they put you on an operating table and did a fake "operation" to replace some part of your body. They showed you the brain or heart they were supposedly putting into you. You were young enough to believe that this was possible. It is not. It was a trick.

What to do about it: Try to explain gently to the young parts that what the abusers said they were doing is actually impossible. If some inside part was watching from outside the body, that part may be able to show you how the trick was done.

44. *Lie*: You were abducted by aliens.

The truth: The people who hurt you in childhood were human beings.

Why they told this lie: They wanted to make sure no one would believe you if you talked about what really happened to you.

How they made you believe it: When you were a child, they drugged and hypnotized you, then people in costumes pretended to be aliens, and took you to a place that looked like a spaceship and abused you there. They might have used films while you were drugged so you thought the things in the films were happening to you.

What to do about it: Recognize that although you may remember something, it might not have been what your abusers said it was. Their abuses are full of tricks and lies, and this was a trick to make your memories appear unreal. Do not let this memory make you stop talking about your other memories.

45. *Lie*: You are a robot, or a computer, or a sex machine, or a killing machine, not a person. Or you have robots inside you who control your mind and body.

The truth: You are a human being, and all your inside parts are parts of that human being.

How they made you believe it: When each part was split off by the abusers' torture, it was told a lie about who or what it was, and the other parts were also told this lie.

What to do about it: Recognize that each part of you, even the ones who have believed they are these things, are human parts, and were created by you, not to serve the abusers but to keep you alive and as safe as possible. Treat the child parts like children, with kindness, and let them begin to play and learn instead of having to do the jobs they were assigned by the abusers.

46. *Lie*: You are a soldier and your duty is to obey without thinking, and never to cry, vomit, show compassion for others, or show soft emotions like fear or sadness.

The truth: It is illegal all over the world for children to be soldiers. When armies make children act as soldiers, they are violating their human rights. You are not, and should not be, a soldier. All emotions are important and positive parts of being human. In case you did not know, you are a human being and part of being human is experiencing and expressing a whole range of emotions, from joy to anger to sadness. Emotions tell us all what is going on inside us and what the truth is.

How they made you believe it: They dressed you up in a uniform and adults in uniforms who called themselves generals or commanders or captains used their power, their size, and their loud voices to frighten you and make you obey. They made you engage in training just like an adult soldier. They might have made you watch films of soldiers marching or fighting. They talked about pride in fighting for their glorious cause, and dying for it. They gave you fake promotions. They shouted at you and told you to obey, not think for yourself. They punished you if you cried, vomited, showed fear or sadness, or showed compassion for others who were being hurt.

What to do about it: Realize that it was not legal for anyone to enslave a child as a soldier. Children need to play and to discover their own interests, not to obey orders unquestioningly. Realize you are now free, and do not have to obey the people who enslaved you as a child.

Allow the parts of you who feel the softer emotions to share with the others, so that your emotions can guide you to the truth.

47. *Lie*: If you fight back against your abusers, you are a traitor and should be punished.

The truth: These people were abusers, and it is right to fight against abuse. If you fought, this showed you were courageous, not a traitor.

How they made you believe it: They punished you whenever you fought against them or refused to do what they told you to do.

What to do about it: Reclaim all the parts of you who fought back, and use their energy now to fight for your healing and to stop child abuse.

48. *Lie*: If you cry or have soft emotions like sadness or compassion, you are weak.

The truth: All emotions are messages to tell you what is going on. Sadness means you have been hurt or suffered a loss; compassion means you care for someone else who is being hurt, and what is happening to them is wrong. Crying is a healthy way to release sad or hurt feelings so you can heal.

How they made you believe it: They punished you severely if you cried or showed emotions like sadness or compassion.

What to do about it: Reclaim your right to cry and to feel what you feel. Recognize that no one will punish you for your feelings now. If any parts of you punish you internally for crying, explain to them that crying is not wrong, that things are different now, and that you will not get into trouble from the abusers if you cry now. Accept and care for the inside parts of you who feel these emotions. Emotions are an important part of your being. Their purpose is to let you know what you need.

49. *Lie*: All parts of you must stay in their assigned "places" in your inner world or structure.

The truth: No one outside your own head knows where your parts are inside, and once you remove parts from their assigned places and move them to places where they can heal, no one outside you will know where they are.

Why they told this lie: They wanted it to be easy for them or future abusers to find each part they had trained.

How they made you believe it: They trained a part of you when you were a very young child with a model of your inner world or structure, to put every part in its place. They told you that everyone must stay in his or her place. They may have punished your parts when they were found somewhere they were not allowed to be. They may have located some parts at certain locations in the body so that a touch on those spots would bring them out.

What to do about it: You can make all kinds of changes to your inner world, and your abusers will never know what changes you have made, as long as no part of you tells them. You can put in healing places, places for play, and places for learning.

50. *Lie*: All parts of you were created only to do the jobs assigned to them by their designers, and if they do not do these jobs they will have no purpose.

The truth: The abusers (who may have called themselves "designers" or "creators" or "manufacturers") did not "create" any of your parts, they only split the existing child into more and more parts by means of abuse, torture, and terror. All of you are parts of one person who was not allowed to develop his or her own interests and abilities.

How they made you believe it: When a part of you was newly split off, that part would not remember what happened to the ones who existed before it, so it believed what the abusers told it about who it was and why it was there, especially because of fear.

What to do about it: Let all your inside parts know that they are human, free them from the jobs they were assigned, and allow them to choose new jobs which reflect their own healthy and positive interests and abilities.

These are some of the most common lies that mind controllers tell their victims. It will empower you to know that they are lies, and you do not have to believe them any longer. Deep down inside you, when you share information and emotions among all your parts, you know the truth. You now have choices that you did not have in childhood. If there are other things your abusers told you, you need to question these things, and consult with your inside parts to discover the truth. As you do this, you will regain your freedom and control of your own life.

SECTION III

BONDS AND BETRAYAL

Why and how they prevent bonding throughout life

Wendy Hoffman

There are two kinds of people in the world—those who have had a mother's love and those who have not.

Having a mother's love seems to be fundamental to having a certain assurance. The expanse of life is so vast and overwhelming that infants need mothers to ease them into it. The deprivation can lead to a long insecurity. Despite the physical pain of torture, degradation, humiliation, being forced to do evil to others—despite all this, being motherless is probably the hardest to bear.

The mother-loved seem to walk through life engulfed in a cloud of being valued and cherished. Those who were deprived of this basic attachment, through no fault of their own, have to fight for self-assurance and to eschew a sense of rootlessness.

Mind controllers have to eliminate the sense of primary attachment in order to gain control of the infant's mind. If the mind controllers are to have the perfect specimen, then they must have a *tabula rasa* (blank slate) from birth or almost from birth. Mind control can be imposed on children and even older children, but infants from multi-generational families are their best bet, because the mind controllers have access to the child from conception, and can prevent the bond that knits together the infant's disparate states.

Bonding permeates all aspects of life, like self-esteem. This essay is about why and how satanic cult perpetrators attempt to prevent its child members from bonding.

Pre-natal and newborn mind control

It is difficult for people to believe that others would deliberately separate children from their mothers physically, emotionally, and spiritually. It is even more difficult to believe that they would start working on fetuses still in the mother's womb. Specific programmers begin the electroshock in the sixth month of pregnancy. They place electrodes on the pregnant woman's skin and thereby blast the fetus. The mother loses contact with the unborn child because of the physical pain on her tender, stretched skin. The programmers have sowed the seeds of an attachment disorder even before the child is born. The effect is somewhat similar to that of the mother who drinks and uses drugs excessively or who becomes seriously ill during the pregnancy. The destructive maneuver of electroshock on the fetus is repeated at intervals throughout the remaining three months of the pregnancy. Persons destined for leadership positions receive this barbaric treatment. Those are the unfortunate individuals the leaders believe must be utterly controlled.

Some mothers, even at young ages, will have insight into the programmers' purpose. Some might even unconsciously remember their own experiences before they were born. Those mothers will stay connected to the child despite the pain. Programmers cannot tell whether the mother has remained connected. Therefore, they cause the infant physical pain after its birth by doing something like pricking its foot. The baby will cry. If it accepts comfort, it is bonded. If it cannot be comforted, it is not bonded. If the infant is bonded, he or she cannot hold a leadership position and might not be allowed to live.

People scheduled to have secondary roles in the cult do not all get this pre-birth torture. But shortly after birth, the perpetrators break the beginning bond with all cult infants. The infants will need comforting in myriad ways and the mothers will be restrained from giving it. A mother will be forced recurrently to starve her baby and render it sleep-deprived. The cult leaders then have the raw material they need, for this child's mind will be far easier to shatter and the child will be more prone to have a trauma relationship with the handler.

Trauma bonds are different from affection bonds. Trauma bonds come from desperation and deprivation, not love and abundance. This first step of deception has been completed. It will be sealed by the time the child is five years old. The emotional pain can shatter the heart. Now the child will have a dissociated brain and a dissociated heart.

In healing from this aspect of this abuse, reach out to these suffering fetuses and newborns within your mind, hold, feed, and comfort them. Tell them you love them. All this is done mentally. Make sure they stay warm and not dehydrated or hungry. Rock and sing to them. Keep them away from mean or toxic people, if possible. Eventually, they will be incorporated into the wholeness of the brain. They have been waiting for the rest of the internal system's acknowledgement all these years.

The bonds between infants and parents, especially mothers, are broken in cult families when infants' emotions are the hottest and most inflexible. While babies are still in their cribs, master programmers set up scenarios to teach them that their mothers do not love or care about them. For example, a handler hurts the child physically, and the mother is forced to walk by the crib without looking at the child who has been starved and is dehydrated and crying. Or the mother feeds a sibling while the starving infant watches.

Children hold on to intense feelings, especially those of rejection and abandonment, which can exist throughout life. When this kind of rejection is repeated often, the child will be wary, reluctant, and later unable, to bond with the mother. Rage then replaces bonding. The drive to be close to people can be strong enough to overcome some of these fearful, angry emotions temporarily, but the fear and anger are likely to surface, along with a conviction that people do not, and will never, care. Survivors might get close to some people, but not thoroughly close. In addition, further programming throughout their lives makes them unable to relax fully with another human being. They can often relate peacefully to animals, however.

All the survivor can do during the healing process is be aware of these parts, talk with them, listen to them, offer them comfort and, if possible, safety from perpetrators. Try to find out, meaning let them or an internal witness tell you how this disruption occurred. You can see your mother as forced to reject you rather than as choosing to reject you, and as a powerless victim trapped in a web of evil, at a time when there were not resources or therapists to help.

In another world, your original mother might have been able to love you. That anger from manufactured rejection can be turned into a healthy self-love, looking to the future while understanding the hideous past.

Cult children are taught how to kill themselves. In case these children do not follow the rules or have minds that cannot be split into pieces, programmers have to arrange for their possible termination. Programmers give mothers the job of helping train their children to attempt suicide. The children are quick to understand that their mothers want them dead. Adah Sachs wrote an article about infanticidal attachment in the book she co-edited, *Forensic Aspects of Dissociative Identity Disorder* (2008). She points out that you cannot switch off bonding. If the parent wants the infant dead, the infant will try to accommodate the parent's wishes, most likely, in an effort to survive. This understanding seals the lack of attachment further. Ironically, mothers might participate in instructing their children to kill themselves in order to save their children's lives. Children who have not mastered the basic rules of cult life are usually expendable. For some survivors, knowing that parents or leaders want them dead is enough to stop suicidal ideations and plans. Why kill yourself because your enemies want you to?

Because life is particularly difficult for survivors, it helps to find one bit of pleasure each day. The pleasure could be in nature, food, animals, hot showers, books, music, sports, and possibly another human, should there be a kind and loving one in your life. Humans who are kind when in their ordinary life personas but not, of course, in their cult personas will not be sufficient. Find a way to allow comfort and pleasure to interrupt the horrors even if the reprieve of pleasure is for a short time.

The sacrificed

Survivors of mind control grow up in a culture that labels some as expendable and disposable. That means their lives are not valued. Leaders can decide when they will die. They can be murdered for disobedience, perhaps for trying to escape, though in general children raised to be expendable do not have the fight left in them to be rebellious. Usually, they are murdered at one of the prescribed ages, such as six or thirteen. Six and sixteen are more common for females; thirteen, eighteen, or thirty-three for males. Their deaths are usually in front of large gatherings—during high-holiday or specially arranged rituals. Some awful lie will be attached to their deaths. For example, children who loved these victims will be taught not to love or those loved ones will be murdered, and other children are told these people were killed because they were traitors, so they should not be a traitor.

It is all orchestrated. Children from birth to about six years old are routinely deprived of love. Then, as if magically, they receive a friend. The cult leaders carefully choose a friend from among their population of sacrificial victims bred for this purpose. Suddenly, for the children who will survive, life is quasi-normal. Someone loves them. There is companionship. They can share with another child and tell their secrets, though they do not know the hidden-life secrets, already well buried and almost irretrievable. Life becomes sweet, worthwhile. They bloom as a person. For about a year. The duration can vary, but at the end of the allotted time, the child who has tasted love is forced to participate in the murder of his or her friend. Naturally, that makes the child afraid to love and guilt-ridden. A particularly compelling account of this cruelty is Stella Katz's "For Miranda," in Alison Miller's *Healing the Unimaginable, Treating Ritual Abuse and Mind Control* (London: Karnac Books, 2012, p. 211).

The mind control message is that love is not allowed, that the cult leaders will murder any person or animal you love. Is this not the worst betrayal, worse even than not knowing your personal history or what your mind is doing at any given moment? To lose the ability to love or to be afraid to love is greater than even losing the ability to think in an organized way because of the mind control and recurrent concussions administered all through childhood to some. To be afraid to love strips people of humanity, even if the fear of loving is to protect beloveds.

If you were born into a criminal mind control type cult, you have to ask whether there is anything in life that is not betrayal.

The victims' mothers grieve. How do you compensate the mothers for what grew in their bodies? The siblings become more insecure. Will it happen to them? Will they be next? What did their sibling do wrong? Why wasn't I nicer? They swim in grief and guilt, as do some of the parents. *What could I have done to protect?* they ask themselves.

This is a world where some are not deemed worthy of life, where freedom counts for nothing. Sadness bursts in this world. People here would have wanted more. If some person or animal known to a cult-raised child becomes ill or injured, or dies, the child is told it is his or her fault. This cements the message that it is not safe to love anyone.

Survivors have to steel themselves; otherwise the loss will eat their leg off. Growing up in an evil world can take away hope. The goodness in these "expendable" victims gave hope to the victims who knew them. Now those victims believe that to love will cause death. Survivors become numb, sometimes only feeling their grief and fear at 3 a.m.

People have different ideas about the afterlife and no one knows for certain. It is possible that the special friend who was murdered young protects you during your life, places a protective shield over your body so that you do not feel the injuries as gravely as you would have otherwise. That has been my experience.

As they live their lives as survivors, some remembering what has occurred, many not knowing—as they proceed with their lives, they notice in themselves a hypersensitivity to loss, abandonment, and rejections. Those who have lost these innocent loved ones carry that pain everywhere. When a fickle friend drops them for the new person on the block, they suffer enormously. When their work is rejected or they are fired, the sting goes deep. The foundation of their lives is loss, and that makes a huge difference to how you develop. The survivors of the "expendables" often gravitate to those who will not live long, who are physically or psychologically vulnerable. It is as if their grief searches for an object. Those with pre-natal programming may find abandonment almost impossible to deal with.

Again, knowing the source of these emotions paves the way for healing them. It was not your fault that your friend was murdered. That murder is not sufficient reason to stop you from loving in the future. The more you understand this, the more you can release unearned guilt and try to relate to others in love. This is not your guilt. It is someone else's.

There is much unrequited love in survivors. That love can be given to yourself as a first act in nurturing yourself back into being who you are and are meant to be. When you are young, you have no way of knowing who you really are, but, as an adult, you can figure it out.

You can take a close look at yourself with the purpose of finding qualities you admire. Forget about surface qualities or even intelligence and talents. Go deeper than genetic gifts. Look at what you have done with yourself to have emerged from this background with humanity, strength and *the ability to think*. Your therapist or supportive friends can help you look deeply into your own soul and pull out the qualities that lead to good self-esteem. There are qualities in everyone that can create self-admiration and a healthy pride. You can learn how to mother yourself. Mothers are meant to make their children feel secure, loved, and capable, with self-esteem the opposite of what happens during mind control preparations.

Survivors, as adults, can do this for themselves.

Good people

In every nook of the world, good people exist. They might be the minority, but they are there. There are rescuers who always have an eye out for how to help people; there are people who grew up in wholesome families and want to share the enormous gift they received of having decent parents; there are benign people with good hearts who want to help everywhere. There are those who admire courage and those who fight to improve and repair the world. There are people who naturally generate wellbeing and love.

Accepting good people into our lives is a challenge for cult torture survivors. We have been programmed to love only our handlers, who control and oversee all aspects of our lives. We do not necessarily love the malicious handlers on our own. We are taught under torture and drugs to transfer our love from a true object such as the child who was sacrificed to the next person assigned to control us. It is no wonder that a handler is often commanded to be a spouse. And when a person from the army of the good enters our lives, we are programmed to reject that person.

Someone good will enter your life when you are a child and an adult and even in old age. This occurrence is an opportunity to find the childhood memory of the one person who loved you in childhood, if you do not have that memory already. You can still bask in that child's love even if they forced you to participate in that soul's death. You tasted love no matter how it ended and no matter that it was prearranged. You know what love is. It can be sifted out from its surrounding tragedies. A good soul touched your life. You were blessed.

The sacrifice certainly constrains the child's ability and willingness to love, but it is not that one-dimensional. The child basked in love for a year. The threat is real, but so is the experience of love's strength.

Children who are programmed not to bond are also placed repeatedly in traumatic situations. Ironically, trauma creates its own kind of intense bonding. War survivors attest to this phenomenon. Their connections to others who share their life-threatening experiences, their sense that only other such survivors can understand, create a bond. Survivors have both an undercoating of not being able to bond and the life experience of extreme bonding—a bonding that untraumatized people probably do not experience and perhaps understand.

Now you might be amazed at what seems to you the fuss normal people make, and, in your opinion, compared to what you have been through, about what seems like nothing much. Remember, however, that normal people think and feel with their whole minds whereas, until you are integrated, experiences in you are encapsulated and felt in only designated sections of the mind. Even small disappointments and hurts are more painful when felt with the whole mind all together.

You can betray your mind control, programmers, handlers, and, unfortunately, your family, know your past and emerge a free person who accepts love and is not programmed to push it away. You can love your child or children. You can finally love yourself. You can stop this dance with betrayal and enter life and become acquainted with freedom and love and with what others consider normal life. They did not have to fight for it with everything in them. You do.

Love becomes a choice. Does one stay paralyzed in fear or go forward to give love to someone else and to receive it? As adults, survivors can go back to those feelings of being afraid to love, see the lies and set-ups and, one hopes, undo the taught and irrational fears.

How they keep you with them

If you were born into a generational criminal mind control cult, your mother might have left you to be sexually abused by other relatives, who may have raped and drugged you; your father might have sold you to scientists who experimented on you; you might have been gang-raped frequently, and you might have been mind-controlled so that you do not know your history or what any one part of your mind is doing at any time. Programmers usurp all aspects of your life and humanity so that you cannot choose a career, or even where to live. They dictate your life and you do not know it because of the mind control these same perpetrators put into you. It does not matter that it is not legal. They have gotten away with it for hundreds of years, and duplicity has increased since families allowed the Nazi scientists and doctors such as Mengele and, now, newer ones to experiment on their children. And currently there is technology to enhance mind control procedures.

Cult children turned adults but still with child parts inside tend to love too much or not enough. They still respond on an infantile level because they have many unhealed, needy infants inside. If they are afraid to love, they may become closed, crisp, withholding adults. If they let their huge infantile need for love be expressed, they will find that partners and friends can never give enough to soothe that need, and they may become ashamed, or blame those who will not or cannot give what a mother should have given years earlier. Then, as they age, they learn to hold back and not give too much, because it will not be reciprocated. Most people have not lived through the heart of evil, or perhaps have had one bad thing happen to them and then strove to avoid any mention of evil in anyone's life. Unlike most normal people, cult people know first-hand what humans are capable of.

From the beginning, survivors have been programmed to believe that their families and cult groups are the only places where they will be accepted. If you come from a cult family and the family members have not healed and are programmed, if you want to be free, it is necessary to leave your family. To leave, survivors have to overcome their fears and this malevolent programming. It might be necessary for them even to abandon younger siblings. The difficulty in bonding makes it easier to leave but it can still be very painful, if not excruciating. Sometimes, a younger sibling will contact the escaped survivor, but the escapee should probably not respond. It could be a setup. The sibling might have been programmed to lure the escapee back home.

Marriage

Many cult marriages are pre-arranged, and people marry other cult victims who also have difficulty bonding. The miseries this abuse causes can seem never-ending. Some cult victims manage to marry a non-cult spouse, and they have a better chance of growing into a close supportive relationship. But the innocent partner will be confused and bewildered and might not be sufficiently protective.

Some people manage to escape their cult families at a young enough age that they can marry unabused mates whom they choose and have children with. They then had a bad beginning but a good ending to their lives, though they will present challenges to their partners through their fear and rage.

As survivors allow themselves to become close to another person, the pain of early disappointments might arise. It helps to have a knowledgeable-about-mind-control, compassionate mate who encourages communication and saying what is held back out of fear. That person can help you break down the walls when your fears become a high tide. You also can drop your mask and be real in that person's presence. As you heal and perhaps bond for real, whirls of pain will swim out of your body. That is the healing process. It interrupts stasis and forces the putrid out. The softness in you that had been frozen can defrost and lead you to the right people. You can feel your heart and mind for the first time.

If you are terrified of bonding with another human, start with an animal. If a dog is too demanding, begin with a cat. Animals can see essentials. They might help you. They know about love, especially if you feed them.

It is unclear whether the deepest fissures in the bonding process can be healed. If people can retrieve the memories of the early programming not to bond, which happens very young, they may be able to heal and erase those scars. Some people can make a commitment to love and even marry. Some need quiet, space around them, and an inordinate amount of solitude to manage the many painful memories each part of their brain is dealing with constantly.

Coming out of this kind of abuse, people often display extremes of behavior. Some become selfish and will do little or nothing for other people. Others work too hard on relationships and/or buy too many gifts for others. Mind control programming forms some of these traits but others are from natural, inherent tendencies. As survivors become healthier, some unhealthy friendships lose their power.

People who have not been loved or properly loved can be hungry and fierce. They can grasp at the possibility of love too hard. Unconsciously, survivors may gravitate to people like their family members. Here is where everyday psychology steps in. Perhaps they want to win over someone with the same deficiencies as their parents or siblings, and make that person more lovable and capable of loving. That is a common and known disaster course. Or, more likely, they were simply mind-controlled to love an undesirable and harmful person.

This kind of prescribed bonding with enemies and simultaneous and consequential pushing away of good people dominate cult members' lives until they untangle the mind control programs and free themselves. You have swung from fierce bonding with enemies to lukewarm bonding with good people. The first part of your life was removed from your control. The second part contains free will. That means you can choose whom to love and even whether to love.

Parenthood

Eventually, children are born to the grief-stricken victim who remains in these criminal cults. Again, that is how cults work. They need something to motivate the victim to be compliant. Having a baby to love ignites the feelings of comfort and security that the original friend brought into the survivor's life. Even a pet can provoke the early knowledge of love. Having a child or pet also creates increased anxiety. You want to protect this being at any cost. You also want to protect your own ability to love.

Many people who cannot bond and cannot love or who overlove can bond to their own newborns. These newborns are often taken away, sometimes the moment they are born. This theft leaves wounds in the mother and child. The leaders of these cults usually leave one child in the biological mother's care, but only so that they have another weapon to control the parent and make her afraid to leave. New mothers sometimes hate their newborns from the moment of their birth, if not before. These mothers realize that their babies will keep them trapped in these mind control cults.

Most survivors unfortunate enough to have had children find it impossible to leave their children or child. They often wait until their children are adults. It is unclear whether it is better for the children if the parent stays in an active cult situation with them. Parents who leave children could possibly return to rescue the children later after they have healed outside this family and cult group. If they stay, they will have to do terrible things to their own children. If they leave, someone else will be forced to do horrible things to these children. The people who keep contact with unsafe family members are usually among those who are re-programmed repeatedly.

Some people leave their families and never really find new families. Families can be insular and not welcoming of newcomers, especially newcomers with such a past. Still, it is far better to be out of a cult family, no matter what the consequences or loneliness. And many people are integrated into other families.

Workplace relationships

The work world can trigger left over feelings from one's family of origin. If bosses and administrators are fair and respectful, they can unknowingly play a strong role in helping survivors heal. They can help teach survivors that people in authority can be just and care about them as individuals. The beginning feelings of the ability to bond can start in a work environment with trust in, and respect for, a boss or supervisor. But if superiors and the overseeing administration are unfair and use people as pawns, for example, overworking and underpaying them while they take the big salaries and bonuses for themselves, or criticizing and micromanaging, then survivors might experience rage and become uncooperative. This kind of work experience can make them rebellious, which is not necessarily bad. If they can object to, and eventually break away from, a disrespectful, hostile work environment, they might eventually be able to break away from programmers, handlers, and abusive families.

When survivors enter the work world, they might automatically treat people who are lazy and not doing their lesser jobs in a cult way, which means abusively and rudely, without even realizing it. The work environment is a place where these actions and attitudes can be brought to awareness promptly and, one hopes, corrected.

Therapy

As survivors grow to want healing, many enter therapy. A major aspect of therapy is learning to bond with your therapist. This is why it is so important for the chosen therapist to be a healthy and wholesome person who does not use people. Survivors have had enough of false bonding with the deficient and sick. There is an element of falsity even with good therapy transferences. A therapist is not seen as a real human being with problems and illnesses like everyone else in the world. It is not a give-and-take relationship. But its one-sidedness can be healing and address the survivor's wounds and deficits in the hothouse type of environment of therapy needed to cure the scars left by grave insults.

The more the bonding issues heal, the freer emerging cult survivors become to have a fuller life, be comfortable with themselves, and become who they were meant to be before the insidious programming and mind control.

When you love, it can hurt your heart, but some pains are worth it. Think of them as birth pains, hard to bear but necessary. We are not really human unless we love. We cannot really parent, or even own a pet, without love in our hearts. It behoves us to undo the programming not to love and join the human race. Grief can overwhelm the human heart, but so can genuine love.

Programmers depend on your remaining unattached and unbonded. Defy them. On the other hand, if you choose to live alone and as a recluse, that is your prerogative and privilege. You deserve to live exactly as you choose.

A drop of color in a glass of water changes the color of the water. Just a drop. I can see from writing about much of my life that my family was trapped under evil. My grandfather was once a scared little boy in Galicia until they forced him to decide to be evil, this grandfather who attempted to destroy so many young minds. My mother was like a firefly closed in a glass jar with only one hole punctured for air. Even when the firefly changed colors fast, it remained lidded and caught. My sister was afraid. My legal father was still a child doing whatever he could not to be a victim. This next generation is under the lid of this oppression. My son and I had a hostile relationship. Now I can see that he was afraid I would be killed, and I was afraid he would be killed, should we show our love. We protected each other by not being close. That's more loving than spending all our holidays together.

I had a year of a boy's love. Sixty years later, I had a friend who nurtured. And another friend who cared enough about me to point me to a therapist who cared that I become free. I had three dogs who loved me. That was all I had. Drops in an expanse but enough to fight the doom that has oppressed my life. A small amount of love can undo what man has contrived for generations, from the beginning of time. Love is that potent.

Family relationships*

Wendy Hoffman

In this whole field of horrendous abuse and evil, the kicker is family relationships. Criminals like the Nazis in Nazi Germany, by contrast, are reputed to have had good family relationships even while they murdered in the cities, towns, and concentration camps. The family relationships in criminal cults, however, are not warm and friendly, except on the surface.

In these families, there are two lives going on simultaneously: the hidden life of tortuous mind control administered in electroshock chairs with drugs and additional forms of torture, secret outdoor and indoor rituals, and inner parts that on command emerge to do an assignment. There is every kind of abuse and emotional, mental, physical, sexual perversion possible. There is also soul-abuse. All that is going on underneath.

On the surface is ordinary life with work and school, family meals, weekends with outings, parties, shopping, films, maybe golf, tennis, or swimming. There's the adults cleaning the house and doing the laundry, the children's sports and music recitals and homework and projects. Cult families do what normal families do in normal life.

* Versions of this essay and the following two were presented at the Survivorship Ritual Abuse and Child Abuse 2016 Conference "Stop Mind Control and Programs", in Oakland, CA.

How do you segue from the worse kind of abuses and torture to an innocent and seemingly normal kind of everyday life? It takes serious mind control starting in infancy not to know the other life. Not only do the abusers usurp your mind and capacity to think and be yourself, they deprive you of a family.

Most survivors of criminal satanic cults do not know how bad their families are. Many idealize them. "I had the best childhood." "My parents loved me." "Life was so peaceful." "My parents cared about me," they say. They recite from their programming to love their families, to idealize their perpetrators.

It is not that they are lying. Some have been trained from birth not to know what is going on, to be blind to reality, not to ever see the whole picture. There are the secret mind control and the innocuous everyday life. Never were the two meant to join hands and live in the light together. There is the family life according to the front person and what society is allowed to see, and life according to the insiders who experienced it.

If there are mind control and torture occurring in what might be called sub-life, this experience has to bleed into everyday life. Parents might have different alters to accomplish hidden cult tasks, but those deeds and feelings resonate in everyday life. The separation between the two lives is never 100%. In addition, some parents will have become "conscious", which means that they will have a partial memory of their secret cult life. They may know consciously how they have treated their children in programming sessions and rituals. Their emotions from one of their roles will leak through into their other roles.

Some relatives are allowed to show kindness, perhaps a grandparent, so that the leaders can threaten to kill that one person if you try to run away, and use that person as someone your inside parts report to about whether you are about to relocate or what you have disclosed to your therapist.

If you have not had adequate family relationships, to recover from this horrendous abuse is to know what your real family life was—perhaps is—like, both the hidden and known parts of it. It is a bit like being a citizen of a country, growing up to believe your country is righteous and fair and discovering later its terrible and criminal abuses of human rights. Organizations created to stop family abuses do not know what happens in these families. Even the victims do not consciously know what occurs in their unfortunate lives.

Incest

Memories of family involvement often start with incest memories. My memories began with bizarre physical abuse—my mother's peeing on me—followed quickly by sexual abuse memories. Incest exists in the normal world, whereas organized criminal abuse with drugs and electroshock usually does not. Incest in cult families can be extensive and involve many relatives. There is also enforced sexual abuse with the family pet. Cult leaders mandate sexual abuse of children for many reasons. They intend to destroy children's self-esteem so that they will start to think of themselves as non-human objects designed to do others' bidding. Incest inserts a rift in family relationships and creates intense jealousy between the incestuous abuser's spouse and the child victim and between siblings. The wronged spouse might take revenge on the child victim, sometimes killing that child or coming close. Incest occurs frequently in families of ordinary life and has similar consequences. But, in cult families, it also begins the preparations for using children as unpaid pornography and prostitution servants for the Mafia groups. Incest teaches these children that their only worth is their use as sex objects. For some satanic criminal cult survivors, there are probably porno flicks floating around the internet today. And snuff porno flicks in which someone is really or supposedly killed.

Children have reporters in them. Those are parts not known to the rest of the internal system. They report everything that happens to them. They can be called out or they can report spontaneously. Parents are told that if they do not sexually abuse their children, their children will be skinned and sacrificed. With the parent watching, the programmers question the children's reporter-parts to ascertain whether they were sexually abused. If the children say they have not been sexually abused, they may or may not be tortured and murdered. The whole thing might be a manipulative lie. But there's no guarantee. Leaders need robots who hate themselves. Parents sexually abuse their children in some cases to save those children's lives. While in a different personality, the same parents might sexually abuse to possess their children and manifest their own hatred.

Love in cult families

Wendy Hoffman

There can be love in these families—deep, genuine, protective love. Here is the love: Some cult parents who are prisoners fight as hard as they can to overcome their mind control, love and protect their children. They have a whole foundational level of destruction within themselves, and still they attempt to be good parents. Surely their children feel the vibrations of that love. Those children may be more loved than even normal children who grow up in ordinary normal families where the parents do not have to fight with everything in them to protect and honor their children. If you are a survivor, you might have had one or two such parents. Or you might be such a parent.

But not all parents are like that. Some, many, children are left with the hidden knowledge that their parents hate and resent them and wish them dead, while, in ordinary life, these same parents go through the motions of being good parents. Unconsciously, children seethe at the hypocrisy.

Love can grow in thick darkness. That love can have the deepest roots. It might not be noticeable, but it is there. It shows when parents mess up a little of their children's programming. When they drop hints about the truth of their lives in normal life. In some cult families, the supposed parent might not be biological. A parent can state in an offhand way who the biological parent is, or whether the child the adult is raising is a biological one.

Those parents might just be blabbermouths, or they might truly want their child to know the truth. They might want their children to know the truth to hurt them, or to help them know reality. For example, my legal father told me who my biological father was. I had thought my legal father was my biological father.

Perhaps the ultimate sign of love is when parents arrange for their children to escape from this criminal world and live far away with a safe family. Cult parents can be like the mother who stood before King Solomon and preferred her child not to be destroyed even if it meant giving up custody of that child. They resemble the parents who lived during the Holocaust and put their children on the transport trains to freedom, not knowing whether they would ever see or find them again and thinking they would not—all so that their children might be safe and live. That's love. Love flourishes in war. Trapped survivors of satanic cult abuse are constantly at war.

Amazingly, love in these cults can also look like leaving your child behind and escaping yourself. The model of escaping into freedom may give a more important message than remaining and suffering and being forced to abuse your children and other people's children. Even grandparents are forced to abuse. I began one of my memoirs with a scene about being forced to abuse my grandchildren.

Family-hunger, planted therapists, and romances

Wendy Hoffman

Some survivors who understand and acknowledge their prior family life, if that family life was horrendous, often remain family-hungry. When you do not have a family for support and love, you are essentially an orphan. Some cult victims are orphans but they do not realize it until they engage in recovery. Many dangers float around the state of being family-hungry. One of the most pernicious dangers of being in this state is the vulnerability to being dominated by cult-planted therapists and handlers. Survivors in general tend to become over-dependent on their therapists. No one else, usually, has heard their stories or understood them. With planted therapists, as with families, two simultaneous relationships exist. There is the everyday, normal life relationship where survivors' front people think the therapist is interested and helping them, and the secret relationship where the insider victims are being closed down, and memories erased from their minds. The hidden relationship is close to murder.

Say you have reported, without your front person's knowledge, to your handler that you are about to have, or are having, significant or break-through memories. From their perspective, you have to be stopped and they will erase your mind to accomplish this. You might get a phone call, probably in the middle of the night or early morning.

This caller will use code words to trigger obedient, robotic inside parts. The caller will call out your memorizers to record the information in your brain and do something like give that part of you a phone number and time to call one of their planted cult therapists, who might not be local. Your front person will know nothing of this conversation. You go to where the voice on the phone tells you to go—to the planted therapist's office.

There might be a hidden black electroshock chair and a team there to program you, depending on their resources and how much of a threat they consider you to be. Then you will be referred to a local planted therapist, medical, Christian, secular, new age, energy specialist—whoever is available and has time in their schedule. The planted therapists are usually paid well, in addition to what they charge you for being mind-controlled. You will end up in what you think is therapy with that person. From there you will have extensive torture sessions to close down any memories of your cult secret life and not to remember that this therapist is a double agent. All while your front person loves and is devoted to the therapist and does not have a clue what is really going on. Your front person will not know that he or she was programmed to love this therapist. But there is one clue. You feel, and possibly journal, chronic anger that never seems to quiet down or resolve. Why should it resolve? This team of double agents is in the process of taking your mind away yet again.

In addition to electroshock, other forms of torture, and drugs, double agents use hand signals, show playing and Tarot cards and other visual cues, and use other nonverbal means and code words to give you close down signals. To the programmed front person, they appear caring and devoted and to give the kind of devotion and acceptance that has not been in your life previously. To the inside parts being worked over, they are vicious and malevolent.

Cult adult survivors long for love, and they also live in normal society in which people get married and start new families. Most marriages are arranged. The two victims usually prefer this marriage to being tortured and murdered. Some marriages occur for social and political reasons and are supposed to look good to the outside world. Some marriages are for punishment, especially if one of the spouses is not obedient enough. Most survivors have handlers to watch them throughout their lives or until they become conscious or trusted. Before marriage, a family member is often the handler. Then the spouse is often the handler. A political leader might have a spouse who is that person's handler. With a spouse as a handler, there is little or no privacy. The handler-spouse does not have to be as bright or ambitious as the watched spouse. The handler-spouse simply needs to know all that goes on in that person's life and know the code words, signals, and triggers that control the victim. The front person of the watched spouse has no idea that the other spouse is a handler. Handler is a new term from military/political circles, and is not necessarily what these cults call this role. There are most likely other, newer terms. Some are made to marry pedophiles who are not cult members. Some cults may allow someone to marry outside their group but keep their affiliations with the group. Other survivors rebel and marry an outsider and get away with it. If a survivor is single, the cult may send a boyfriend or girlfriend—or even just a friend—to get close to the survivor and become the handler.

And so we may be left in a family-hungry state, craving family love, thinking we love our perpetrator families, being bonded to enemies, and hating ourselves and not knowing why our lives turned out so awful. This is all mind control.

Therapists' responses to survivors: countertransference and attunement

Alison Miller

I would like to separate out some particular kinds of responses which are common in therapists treating survivors of extreme and organized abuse. If you are a therapist, you may recognize some of these in yourself, and if you are a client, you may recognize them in your present or past therapist.

Part 1: Countertransference

The term "transference" refers to the way in which a client may project to a therapist things from a previous relationship, for example with a parent. Therapists are expected to recognize this, and gently help the client see what is going on without taking it personally.

A related term, "countertransference," has been used to mean many things, but its primary meaning has been a therapist's reaction to a client's transference. I am going to tell you a story regarding my experience with one client, whom I only saw once for an extended session. I do not know whether she had been victimized by an organized group; if she had, she was not aware of it. But the way she treated me illustrates a very strong negative transference, and my response shows my countertransference.

The abusive client

She called several times over a period of weeks. She was seeking a therapist for early childhood trauma. She was living on a disability pension because her trauma history made her unable to function. She now spent all day, every day, writing about her suffering. Each message said that she was "in a regressed state" when she called. She did not know whether or not to come and see me. We swapped messages for a while. She had a lot of questions for me about how I worked. I offered to see her for half price. One time she reached me, asked a couple of her questions, and made an appointment. Then she cancelled it, saying she had more questions. Eventually, I suggested she come in for a free meeting in which she could ask her questions face to face, and she agreed to do this, and showed up.

She said she'd been in therapy for thirteen years with various therapists. Some of them had triggered her into continuous flashbacks by going into the trauma prematurely. Others had given her advice she was unable to follow, which did not feel realistic for her, such as to go for a walk every day. One had "feelings" for her but kept on seeing her for years after acknowledging this. One of the therapists had worked with her inner child parts, but she had been upset that he talked with the parts and not with her, even though she was present for these conversations. Her most recent therapist had been a wonderful, gentle woman who had discontinued working with her because her neediness had triggered the therapist's own trauma.

As I listened to her talk about the previous therapists, I began to be seduced into seeing all the mistakes they had made, and believing I could, of course, do better than they had. I would be the savior that no one else had been. Though I would not make any of the mistakes they had made. Oh yes, all my years of experience had paid off and I would avoid all these traps.

She stated that she had a lot of trauma about being controlled and disempowered. And she had many young parts that she had to control. She had names for all her "thought patterns" but she did not know whether or not those were the parts. I suggested she think this question in her head, and see whether she would get an answer. She reacted immediately. I was telling her what to do. I said I did not intend that, just a mild suggestion of something she could try if she liked. "Now you're trying to make me feel guilty."

We returned to the parts. She said there was a critic who held imaginary conversations with other people. "You must be thinking I'm very difficult to work with." I asked why she said that. "Because I'm so complicated, because I've had so many bad experiences and I do not trust anybody." She said that besides the early abuse by her father, who lived with her and her mother until she was three, she had a whole childhood of emotional abuse by a controlling mother, who told her what she thought and felt and believed and would do with her life. She explained that her mother's constant control and criticism made her have a constant inner commentary about whomever she was talking with.

I asked what the commentary had said about me. "You were trying to control me when you told me to think a question in my head and listen for the answer." "Your tone of voice on the phone message when you said I should press '1' sounded very bossy." After she came up with each interpretation of my behavior, I would explain it, and she would seem to accept my explanation. We would talk a little more about her and her prior experiences (mostly of therapy). I saw a hurt childish expression on her face, followed immediately by a skeptical expression. "Do you have a protector part around?" "No, I was having thoughts about what you said." "What thoughts?" "I thought you were trying to make me feel guilty." It went on like this. I said "I saw a skeptical expression on your face again. What were you thinking?" "How do you know I was skeptical? Now you're telling *me* what *I* think."

I disclosed that I had had a very critical husband, who would tell me his interpretation of my motives and then refuse to hear my explanation. It was like throwing gasoline on the fire. Aha! I had disclosed an area of vulnerability. I could be hurt by people imputing nasty motives to me. I "hadn't worked through my stuff," as she put it. She was yearning for a therapist who had worked through their stuff so thoroughly that nothing she did could upset them. She was the client, they were the therapists. I suggested that statements about how she felt when I said or did any particular thing would be preferable to her telling me what she thought my motives were. No, she was a survivor of child abuse, so she was entitled to behave any way she liked, she could not help it, and any therapist worth their salt had to be strong enough not to be upset by it.

Time went by. I began to feel sucked into a vortex. An old, familiar feeling, which nothing but a divorce had been sufficient to get rid of. No, I wasn't just "getting triggered." It was being done to me. She wanted to take out on a therapist all the anger she had at her mother by treating someone the way her mother had treated her. And any therapist with a messiah complex (which most of us have a bit of) would be seduced into trying to master the situation, work through the transference and countertransference, and would eventually fail. I began to realize why there were so many notches on her gun.

. . . "Well," I finally said, "I do not see how we're going to be able to get through this. I do not have a solution. I cannot work with someone who keeps 'mind-reading,' making statements about my motives, telling me that I'm trying to control or manipulate or induce guilt. And you cannot just make statements about how you feel in relation to my behavior; you need to describe the bad motives you assume I have. I cannot imagine conducting therapy in which I am having to monitor every move and every facial expression so that it doesn't make you think I'm trying to do the things your mother did. Mind-reading is intrusive, and if you cannot or will not stop yourself doing it, I guess I cannot work with you. That's enough; I'm tired." I stood up. It had been two and a half hours, on a day that I'd been going to have off.

She sat there stunned for several minutes. This is not how it was supposed to go. I was supposed to face my challenges and try to work with her, see my own inadequacies and self-deceptions in the process, and let her continue to accuse me of all those things and try to provoke me into doing all those things, while I tried desperately to keep my cool. And instead I said that I would not work with her. She sat there for a while waiting for me to change my mind. I started to pack up. Finally, she said, "Can you suggest another therapist?" I thought about it. "No, I cannot," I said. "You need someone who's less sensitive." "You mean *more* sensitive," she said. "No, I mean *less* sensitive. Someone who won't get hurt when they're continuously accused of unkind motives . . . But the problem is, any therapists I know who are that insensitive are also egotistical and controlling, and you've said you do not like those things. So I really cannot think of someone to recommend." She did not know what to say. She left meekly, saying "Thank you for your time" as she went out the door.

I hoped she'd write about it for a good week or two, trying to figure out what happened. Maybe she would learn something. I did. I learned to recognize and refuse an invitation to be abused.

Maybe what this woman was doing was "projective identification"—trying to make me feel as bad as her mother had made her feel. Or maybe she was a victim of mind control who had programming to exhaust or burn out a therapist. Looking at her history of therapists, it could have been either. But I did not see a genuine desire to learn from another person, a recognition that I was trying to help her, or a desire for change.

We therapists have to be wary of being sucked into the invitation to be the great helper who can help when no one else can; in this example, I fell into that trap. We also have to notice our own feelings in response to the client in order to determine whether or not this can be an effective therapeutic relationship. In this case, my own feelings let me know that it would not work to see this client.

Transference and countertransference happen all the time, even within a good therapeutic relationship. During the year that Wendy lived in my city and we engaged in long therapy sessions three times a week, there were a few occasions when she became irrationally angry with me. On one occasion, I recognized that her irrational anger was related to some of her inside parts, but I assumed it was the group of parts we had just discovered. It was not. The big one came on a Friday. I commented on something in the news about Israel. Wendy became infuriated and accused me of being anti-Semitic. It was an absurd accusation, given our history together. I pointed that out, trying to show her the obvious, that if I had been anti-Semitic, we would not have been able to do the work we did together. But she persisted in attacking me about it. While I had no fear of her being physically violent with me, her fury aimed at me felt like a tear-gas assault. This could have alerted me to something very important, but I was too dense to catch on, because I was hurt by the unfair attack. My own past experiences with someone angry at me who became violent had made me very sensitive to blame, and I recoiled at the force of her anger and blame. I asked her to please not attack me in this way. Wendy cut the session short and went home angry. On the weekend, I called her to ask whether she was coming to our Monday session, and she snapped at me nastily, "Of course."

What survivors say to their therapists on the first level is often what they are programmed to say. Underneath that is the story of how they were programmed to say it. If we therapists can recognize when someone is speaking from a program, we can search for the training that made them say such things. In this case, I missed it because I was so offended by Wendy's accusations.

After I asked her to, Wendy held in her irrational anger at me, and stopped writing about it in the journal entries she sent me. What I did not know was that these attacks resulted from current abuse. Perpetrator group leaders (both Illuminati and Nazis) from the east had flown to town and abused her, including (of course) injecting her with what was probably an amphetamine to make her angry, assaulting her painfully, and telling her it was all my fault. Dissociated anger is already violent when it comes out, disconnected from the rational parts of the person; the drug added to that. They wanted her to pick a fight with me. Neither most of Wendy nor I was aware of the current abuse, and we often wondered together why she had not been pursued. The pursuers had accessed a very separate part of her personality system through well-hidden parts, who did not know me. The manufactured feelings against me from those parts, feelings that belonged to the perpetrators, were leaking through. But because, in my countertransference, I shut down her anger expression, we did not access the information about what was happening. Perhaps we would not have anyway, but we will never know. If we had found out about the current abuse, we would have known that the perpetrators were aware of when she had to leave Canada, and would have been suspicious of the American people who offered to help with that. It might have protected Wendy from a great deal more pain.

The therapist's own transference

All therapists are human beings, and our reactions to people are formed on the basis of other people we have known. Over the years, an experienced therapist learns to pay attention to any personal overreactions and deal with their sources, so that they do not contaminate the relationship with the client. In the story of the abusive client, I did notice a reaction of mine based on her similarity to someone who had judged and criticized me in the past. This in itself was not enough to make me conclude I would not be able to work with this person. The fact that I consciously recognized the similarity actually made me less vulnerable to a transference that would make me assume she was exactly like him when she was not.

But we therapists, like anyone else, are susceptible to projecting our own issues and past experiences on our clients. If you are a client and you find your therapist consistently reacting to you inappropriately, you need to pay attention to this. If you bring it to your therapist's attention, and he or she does not take responsibility for it, it is time to find a different therapist. You are not going to therapy in order to have to deal with the therapist's own issues. Some therapists are unhealed from their own pasts. And some are dangerous cult plants.

Part 2: Attunement

Falling in maternal love with a client

There is a phenomenon I have experienced personally, and which I have witnessed in several therapists over the years working with those severely abused as children. I think of it as "falling in maternal love" with our abused clients. Mothers fall in love with their newborn children. That love combines delight in the infant with an intense desire to protect that baby from all possible harm. An article by Chris Woolston, "The science behind love and mother–infant bonding" (https://consumer.healthday.com), explains how this kind of love is biologically hard-wired into us. The sight of our own infant, or the sense of its prenatal presence, stimulates a hormone, oxytocin, which gives us a feeling of intense love. We are fascinated by the baby, and at the same time fiercely protective of him or her. Even men experience this. And the baby falls in love with you, too. I remember how strongly this love hit me when I had each of my own children. It went far beyond anything I had experienced in romantic love.

Any multiple, especially a survivor of mind control and ritual abuse, is full of unloved infant parts, who long for the nurturance they never received when the body was an infant. Those parts do not really understand that they live in an adult body, and that no one can be with them twenty-four hours a day and protect them from all harm.

When I met my first survivors of ritual abuse and mind control, about whom I wrote in the first chapter of *Healing the Unimaginable,* I was both shocked and fascinated. And I fell in love, maternal love. They were little children within adult bodies, little kids who had gone through experiences far beyond my imagining and beyond anything I had read about or seen on television. They were, in their thinking and behavior, clearly still young children, stopped in their growth by those experiences while the body continued to mature. Two other members of my team at the Mental Health Center also had their first multiple clients, not ritual abuse survivors, but still survivors of extreme abuse, with tortured child parts inside, and they, too, fell in maternal love with their clients. I think it is a biological, hormonal response to the helpless infant in need of protection.

Those were the days of unorthodox family therapy interventions, where it was acceptable to see clients outside the office, and I visited my clients' apartments and took them on outings that their child insiders would enjoy. Somehow, I just wanted to make it up to them for everything they had gone through.

Of course, I was unable to keep up this intensity of relationship. I had to stop the outings when I discovered that my impersonator within the cult was taking advantage of it to take them out to bad places, pretending to be me. I learned of the safety provided by the structured office setting (with a good alarm system). One of my clients kept getting me mixed up with his mother, as a result of cult interventions involving the mother and my impersonator. The feeling of being "in maternal love" with my clients with little children inside gradually wore off, and was replaced by weariness and anxiety. I began to realize quite quickly that even though I felt this love for my clients, I could not keep them safe from harm and I could not give them the attention and caring that they had never received in childhood.

As I moved into private practice, the word went around town that I worked with multiples, and other therapists quickly offloaded such clients onto me. Several of the next survivors I saw came from therapists who had dumped them after becoming overinvolved. One pastor therapist was told by his wife that he could not keep spending all those extra hours with this other woman (who was frequently a little girl). There was no sexual involvement; it was maternal, or perhaps paternal, love. Another therapist mistook his feelings for his attractive client for romantic love, and assumed she felt the same way when her young child alters wanted to be close to him and feel the love they had never experienced. His abandonment of her was deeply traumatizing, and her eventual realization of what he believed was going on just as traumatic. One woman therapist was overwhelmed by dozens of daily emails from her client (resulting from programming to "burn out the therapist"), and eventually dumped the client after a serious suicide attempt ten years into therapy. Each of these therapists made promises to a client that he, and she, could not possibly keep. Then the client was brutally let down. Each of these clients made good progress when my love for them and contact with them were held within safe and consistent boundaries.

My friend who directs a counselling center for refugees tells me that her supervisees frequently become overinvolved with their clients out of this maternal love, the desire to help the wounded and protect them from further harm.

I have seen this maternal love in several therapists to whom I have provided online consultations. They become totally overinvolved with their first multiple client. They try to protect that client from all harm, something that no therapist can do. Their maternal protection takes the place of the adult self-protection that the client needs to develop. It cannot be sustained. We cannot be our clients' mothers. They have to find parts inside who can mother the younger ones. If they do not have a real mother, they have to accept that reality and grieve that loss rather than looking for a replacement. Therapists, watch that you do not respond to your clients' needy and abandoned infant parts by extending yourself further than you can manage or is good for the clients. If you do this, you will end up abandoning them.

When we work with adult or adolescent survivors of child abuse and neglect, we have to help them develop their own inner resources, rather than letting our maternal love lead us to become their leaning posts and to promise them the mothering they never received.

The attuned therapist

The attuned therapist feels his or her client's feelings, without being overwhelmed by them. It is much like what happens in a healthy relationship between mother and child, an attunement that allows the child to be understood and to grow up gradually. Siegel, in *The Developing Mind*, 2012, p. 69) says:

> For "full" emotional communication, one person needs to allow his state of mind to be influenced by that of the other . . . the therapist's sensitivity to the patient's array of signals allows his own state to become aligned with that of the patient . . . The alignment of the therapist's state allows him to have an experience as close as possible to what the patient's subjective world is like at that moment . . . Such an alignment permits a nonverbal form of communication to the patient that she is being "understood" in the deepest sense.

I can often tell what a client is going through by tuning in to what my own body is feeling. I imagine myself holding the client's feelings within my chest, close to my heart, with a thin but strong barrier between her feelings and my own, so I can tell which is which. This attunement is crucial for a good therapeutic connection. Wendy told me that I was particularly attuned to her very young infant parts; she described it as "the therapist's heart coating the heart of the newborn infant."

Siegel says that the need for nonverbal attunement persists throughout life, and is essential to intimate relationships. He states,

> Even at a physical distance, one mind can directly influence the activity—and development—of another through the transfer of energy and information. This joining process occurs via both verbal and nonverbal behavioral responses, which function as signals sent from one mind to another. (2012, p. 277)

I think that possibly "psychic" awareness of other people's emotional states may be a part of this. When a mother is aware of her connection to her unborn child, it is not through verbal, visible, or audible signals. In my childhood and teens, I experimented with telepathy with my siblings and friends. I discovered that my ability to sense what someone was thinking was most accurate when we communicated mentally about something with emotional content, like choosing one of the people we knew who had been at a particular event, rather than letters or numbers or symbols.

As we therapists work with clients who quite frequently have been trained in what are considered paranormal or spiritual abilities, or who have resorted to using such abilities for self-protection, we need to develop an understanding of such abilities. I updated myself on the research about parapsychology (Carter, 2012) and discovered that such natural (though poorly understood) abilities are widespread among humans and also animals, but are generally quite weak and not necessarily very accurate.

One of my dissociative clients had a five-year-old part who had developed her ability to do something she called "seeing the colors." She would stare at the area around my head for a long time. She eventually explained that she saw colors there that showed whether a person was good or bad, and until me she had never been close to anyone who was not bad. I presume she was looking at what some people call the aura. This little inside girl took it upon herself to train me in becoming aware of what the parts in her system were remembering or thinking, because they were unable to talk about it. She actually expected me to read their minds. She wanted me to sit quietly with whatever part came out, tune in to whatever was going on in her head, then put forward a tentative hypothesis based on my own sense of what parts were around and what they might be remembering. Having been trained not to do suggestive therapy, I was reluctant, but this seemed to be the only way to work with this client, at least in the early stages of therapy; otherwise we could spend over an hour in complete silence. If nothing came to me, she would encourage me to "reach in." Sometimes I would get a picture in my head, sometimes emotions. I discovered that these very young parts would correct me if my perception was not quite right, although they did not understand that I was not actually in their head, and did not get why I could not just walk in and rescue trapped internal children. Now they are able to tell me things without my having to guess, but their training paid off in my ability to sense what is going on in a client. I have had numerous experiences of sensing what is in a client's mind. I can sense whether other alters are listening, what emotions they have, whether they have questions or are making internal comments, and what they need from me. I not only feel my clients' feelings, but I sometimes see what they are seeing internally, or become aware of an answer (e.g., a name) which they are not telling me. I dreamed Wendy's internal structure in which her hidden parts used to live shortly after I began working with her, when she did not know the structure. It was such a vivid and bizarre dream that I knew it did not belong to my own life. If I have a significant dream relating to my life, I usually know what it is about. I told Wendy my dream in case it had significance for her, and she gasped and told me what it was about.

If we therapists can make use of such abilities, it can help in our work, but we have to be aware of how easy it is to be misled by a felt sense of something that might be inaccurate or a projection of our own. Attunement can actually help us get a sense of what is in a client's head.

Survivors and therapists, if you have ability or training in these abilities, do not dismiss them as "satanic," but also do not rely on them as if they are unfailingly accurate, because they are not. Instead, use them to form tentative hypotheses about what might be going on in others, then use regular methods to discern whether these are accurate.

SECTION IV

THE HORRORS OF THE ABUSE

Therapists and horror*

Alison Miller

In 1990, I plunged with fascination into work with my first clients who exhibited dissociative disorders, feeling that at last I was doing "real psychology." Perhaps because I worked with children and adolescents as well as adults, it was relatively easy for me to catch on to the personality switches, and adapt my conversational style and therapy technique to the age of the part of the person who was presenting at the time. What I was not prepared for was the horror of what these people had experienced, and which some of them were still experiencing, as the abuser group that considered them its property was still active. At the time, I wrote in my personal journal,

> I have a reservoir of pain—a head full of horrors—from my clients. I have gone through incredible suffering with people. I have not only listened to them tell about past traumatic events, I have watched them abreact them and used my intuitive awareness of their feelings as a guide to what they are going through. I have watched adults experiencing themselves as infants being choked, electroshocked, subjected to terrible pain, having sharp things poked in them, being smothered

* The first part of this work was published in *Therapy Today* in April 2016.

> with pillows, having baby bottles and penises rammed down their throats, drowning in semen, drowning in pools and swamps, being beaten up with limbs broken, being tortured with unbearable pain such as nerve gas, and being raped in every way imaginable. I have been their link to safe present reality as they relive these experiences. I have also had to tune into their terror as they watch other people being tortured and killed in slow, agonizing ways, and are told that if they talk about it or are "traitors" this will happen to them. I have also had to deal with clients' memories of such things that have just happened, within a day or two of when we abreact them. I have had to cope with knowing people are not safe in their apartments or on the street, because evildoers can and do abduct them against their will and do these things to them. I have had to cope with not only death threats to my clients, me, and our families, but also with detailed and explicit descriptions of how those murders will be carried out.

I listed many more abuses than the ones I have reported here. I remember the sense of isolation and the feeling of being overwhelmed. I also remember, however, the satisfaction of giving these survivors their first real connection with a safe, caring person who was not part of the world of torturers. Even when some of them were punished with rape and torture for disclosures to me, they kept coming back. And I began to see improvement in many of them.

The sense of overwhelm and being plunged into horror wears off somehow. You get used to it. I do not know whether I dissociate those emotions, or if I just have accepted that these unimaginable things happen, so I need to pull up my socks and get to work on dealing with them, as you would in rebuilding after an earthquake. I know that I can now hear such things without flinching, which is important as survivors test you out to see what you can stand. One survivor described his therapist to me as "too squishy"—meaning too easily affected by what he might want to disclose. With time, you become less squishy.

Someone needs to work with these clients, not just out of compassion but because it is through them that the truth becomes known and the abuse stopped. My books are full of survivors' own stories, as is my client Wendy Hoffman's memoirs, *The Enslaved Queen* (2014) and *White Witch in a Black Robe* (2016a). The power to tell one's own story is the power to regain one's life. You can help give this power back to the most abused of humanity. Your biggest asset in this work is not your knowledge; it is your ability to form a solid therapeutic relationship (empathy, warmth, and genuineness). You learn from experience. However, it saves a great deal of time if you have already learned about these abuses and structured personality systems, so that your client does not have to teach you everything.

I recently moved to a very friendly neighborhood of retired people, and when my neighbors held a welcome party for me I managed to tell them that I worked with survivors of the most severe child abuse, and consulted to other therapists doing this work. Someone said something like, "Isn't that upsetting to you?" I lamely said, "Someone has to do it," and another person changed the subject. The question seemed to be "Why would anyone do work that exposes them to horror and pain?" Well, one reason could be that it could have been you who had these experiences, but it was not, and that is not because you are any better than those who went through such things.

On a single day, I consulted to two therapists. The first, a Christian, had been listening to a fourteen-year-old part of her ritually abused client talking about a very traumatic experience. Overwhelmed by the horror and sadness of the client, the therapist suggested a guardian angel might be there for the fourteen-year-old. The client's response was "There were no angels, *ever*, not at birth, not in this situation." The therapist proceeded to suggest that maybe someday they could let angels be there. The result was that another part came out and did an incantation. The therapist compounded the problem by asking whether this was to send away anything good, and was surprised when the client's protector part became understandably angry. The client sent an email saying just "I HATE ME."

What was this therapist doing? I think she was defending herself against the terrifying challenge to her worldview. The reality that the client had felt completely abandoned by all forces of good was frightening to her. No wonder. I pointed out that she was invalidating the client's feelings and experience, and, furthermore, she was feeding in to the client's perpetrator-induced belief that she as a child was so evil that God would not help her, and her own incantation had the power to drive away God or angels. This well-meaning therapist had taken on this survivor with complete faith in her interventionist God's ability and desire to relieve the client's pain, and now her faith was shaken.

The second therapist, a Jungian, was older and much more experienced than the first. But she constantly went into despair about her ritually abused client, whose functioning had deteriorated, probably as a result of re-traumatization by the local cult group. She admitted to me that she dreaded seeing the client, though when with her she felt a very deep compassion. She was aware that the despair she was experiencing was also how her client felt, and she was also aware that her worldview had changed as a result of working with this client. She did not want to take on another such client, and given her age, it would have been unwise in any case. When I suggested to her that her recoil reaction might be a reaction to evil rather than to the client herself, this made sense to her. She would have liked me to produce some wonderful thing to help her have hope for her client, but the only thing I could say was that often a survivor's apparent getting worse was just a result of the cult-loyal parts of the client doing their jobs, and I did not believe that all her steadfast caring had gone to waste.

It is inevitable that clients who have experienced ritual abuse or mind control will challenge the worldview of any therapist or other helper. We all have to come to grips with "Where was God?" "How can human beings engage in such deliberate evil?" and "What kind of a world is this?" And there are no easy answers. Yet, we cannot turn our backs on those who have experienced these evils. That is what most of Europe did during the Nazi occupation, and the result was the Holocaust. We have to grapple with the unanswerable questions and make sense of them. We have to avoid giving easy answers to our clients, and constantly check ourselves to see whether our fear is being communicated to our clients, who are exquisitely sensitive to people's inability to hear their real experiences. It is our loving presence, not our glib explanations, that will let them know that there is love in the world, and that some people choose good, and do not turn their backs on those harmed by evil.

Therapists, you will be unable to hide your feelings from your clients, but it is important that you process them in private, even if it leads to significant changes in your view of the world. You can tell your survivor clients that it is not them you are reacting to, it is the evil of what was done to them. Some will not be appeased by your saying this.

Survivors, if you see shock and horror in your therapist when you first talk about some of your experiences, this does not necessarily mean that your therapist will not be able to handle what you must deal with. It does mean that he or she is having to come to grips with some realities you have known about for a long time. It does not mean your therapist hates you, just because he or she hates what you have gone through. Try to be generous and patient with your naïve therapist.

The purpose of infant torture

Wendy Hoffman

Infant torture has not received sufficient attention. Not enough victims remember it, or people think it is too gruesome to deal with. Some of the early *exposés* of mind control and the creation of programmed slaves, such as the film *The Manchurian Candidate,* avoid infancy completely. *Manchurian Candidate* is a quasi-fictionalized version of mind control, but this omission is still important.

Perpetrators have to get their hands on infants. For the more strenuous assigned roles, they start in the womb. The programmed newborn is essential for the continuation of these criminal groups. First of all, the child has to be born unbonded, and to remain so. (See "Why and how they prevent bonding" (pp. 75–88.) Then, once a child is born, very serious training starts full blast without interruption. Perpetrators, usually family members whose job in ordinary life would be to love, believe they have to give the unambiguous message to newborns that they are toys, objects, possessions, if these criminal cults are to continue to exist. They set out to overwhelm unattached newborns and do it through torture. They erase any remnant of a soul that may have lingered. As long as they can keep these poor beings away from any source of love, they have a good chance of succeeding. Apparently, you need someone giving and not just taking to let a sense of self flourish. The sense of self is even more delicate and fragile than orchids or creativity. But the human soul is resilient.

How do you torture a newborn? you may ask. Even newborns in ordinary life are tortured. They often die as a result. Torture for criminal cult newborns, however, is more regulated and not a passion crime. There might be some out-of-control torture in these hidden cults but that style of torture is an aberration and not endorsed. It can happen, though, because some programmers are driven insane. But how do these criminal organizations torture their future leaders as newborns? The same way they torture children, older children, teenagers, and adults. The only difference is that newborns cannot yet be seated in electroshock chairs.

As a newborn, you would be placed in a carrier, set perhaps on a dining room or kitchen table. There may be a support under your flimsy neck. You have not been fed or given a drink for many hours, a lifetime for an infant. The underlying landscape of cult victims is hunger and dehydration—both essential for creating a mind-controlled slave. You spend much of your infant time sucking on air. You are longing to be touched and held and someone might start massaging, say, your feet. Soon this same person inserts needles between your tiny toes. You are introduced to the combination of pleasure and pain and pleasure followed swiftly by pain, which will become a life theme. This programmer is not the only person present. Other adults surround the two of you. The programmer is often a relative in ordinary life or family friend, rarely a stranger. In rural districts, a stranger might stop by periodically to supervise. Needles go into other parts of your trembling body. If you begin to cry, a pillow goes over your face to almost suffocate you. You are not allowed to release feelings, which crying can accomplish. It is difficult to believe, but the programmer places a metal head vise around your malleable skull. It feels sharp, digs in, cuts. The programmer tightens and releases, tightens and releases the vise as he moves his giant lips and says words. You do not understand the words, of course, but some part of your brain memorizes them. Later, when you have achieved formal language, that part will translate from sound to words what was said to you. It is usually something like this: "You are our possession. We own you. You will do whatever we say. You are not free. You will never be free. You belong to us." This message in words is one aspect of programming.

Programmers also use hand signals. The infant cannot understand them but some part inside will memorize the movements and translate them later in life. They are being sensitized to watching hands for messages. Colors, tarot and playing cards, pictures of containers that split off parts will be placed in later are also present.

My programmer also strangled and shook me as a newborn and must have done something like break or dislodge my neck. He molded it back together since his goal was not to murder me.

Programmers also shoot tasers along the sides of the infant's body. Some of the electricity may make infants who had been programmed in the womb remember its former use. They are stunned by the tasers. In addition, programmers spin the newborns on a plank with a neck support. The consequential dizziness also overwhelms the poor human being and makes him or her lose any grip on life or reality and certainly any belief in the self's ability.

The stretching begins now to render the newborn a satisfactory sexual slave. Fingers go into the mouth, rectum, and, for females, vagina. The stretching that renders infants rapeable creatures in programmers' opinion has begun. Even chronically raped people can have touch deprivation.

A good example of how programmers overwhelm these unformed, unloved beings is their trainings to pee on command. When I told Alison, my enlightened therapist, that cult children have to control their pee before the age of six months, she did not believe it was possible. But Alice Miller (1983, 1997, p. 88) writes about German mothers with a compulsion for cleanliness teaching their newborns not to wet or dirty their diapers by the age of six months.

If a cult baby wets, the programmer slaps and beats the infant, punching it in the stomach. This happens over and over again. The sharp infant figures it out after months of being hurt. The duller ones just get hit continuously. Either way the programmer wins. This is another example of the infant's being overwhelmed and taught that it has no power, no rights, no entitlement, no human dignity that would be a natural response to early life. It is helpful if survivors find these infant parts who were prematurely toilet trained, to reduce their despair.

Newborns might or might not have a concept of death. If they do, they would want to die. At least they want to go away. This underlying coating of not wanting to be alive or to be here stays with them on some level throughout life, perhaps until they are fully healed.

From pre-birth to birth to after birth, this is the message, this is the rule. The torture and lack of caring produce the kind of pain that eats away bones. These infant feelings form an unrelenting sack placed under the solar plexus that can follow the survivor throughout life, unless they locate these parts, rescue, and heal them.

In Illuminati programming, the thirteen splits formed are accomplished by the victims' sixth month of life. They are separated and placed in containers. For me, it was a coffin. The containers are sealed and placed below the structure that has yet to be built internally, starting at three years old. These containers below the structure will feed the subsequent structures with feelings of hopelessness and despair. If survivors are ever unfortunate enough to be under the influence of close-down specialists who want to reignite programming and keep them slaves, those close-down specialists will make their way to this structure and try to make sure the designated newborns and infants stay in their sealed containers.

During all this early torture, it is most likely that there will be some natural splits. Even without the torture, the heartbreak, sadness, fear, anger, and loneliness the infants experience are enough to cause a shredding of the personality system.

As the months go on, programmers will do all they can to cement these splits. They will color-code them and assign them visual cues and hand signals. They have the foundation of a highly programmable slave.

The hunger, dehydration, and torture destroy the will. But, apparently, it has not been completely destroyed, because so many victims are becoming free, telling their stories, and emerging as true survivors. They are overcoming their infancy.

More good news is that there are cracks. Sometimes programmers deliberately and secretly leave in cracks. Other times the cracks come from programmer incompetence. The times are ripe for those cracks to open wide. I hope all the people who died slaves can hear. We are making our way toward freedom.

Spinning

Wendy Hoffman

Years after a cult "therapist" was hired to close down my recovery process, years after I had been living like an empty shell, a mindless robot, the memories began to fight their way to the surface. As they tried to creep out, episodes of dizziness assaulted me. I would hold onto my bed and try to steady myself. I had to wait a long time until the feeling that I was being spun round and round subsided before I could start my day or even get out of bed. I clung to the mattress. The feeling became more intense as the weeks went by. I went to my doctor, who referred me to a neurologist, who ordered thousands of dollars' worth of MRIs and MRAs. They revealed nothing to account for the feeling of intense spinning. I did not even know that I could call it a feeling of intense spinning. I thought it was merely dizziness without a known cause.

After every programming session, the programmers spin most infant, child, adolescent, or adult victims in electroshock chairs, in rotatable floor chairs, or on spinning boards. They have spinning boards for infants. The spinning is meant to be a barricade to keep you from knowing what happened to you. Programmers feel that their victims will not be able to quiet the spinning and thereby reach the harrowing memory.

I did not need a neurological workup. I needed to quiet the spinning so that I could discern the programming to feel spinning and also what lay underneath it.

The most effective way to stop the feeling of spinning and the memory of having been spun is to find the part whose job is to release these sensations should the memory become close to consciousness. This is not the part that holds the sensations and memories but, rather, the part that floods the victim when the victim comes too close to knowledge. The part who allows the dizziness to overtake the victim is not dizzy but has the control to get other parts to release dizziness. That part is like a conductor of an orchestra. He calls out the musicians who play instruments but does not play an instrument him or herself. Reassure, reason with, and educate that part. This feeling comes from an event in the past (unless the event just happened). The extreme dizziness in the present results from this part doing his or her job to cover over the memory and block it with this distraction. Talk to this part about the benefits of healing and freedom.

The spinning also spreads the feeling or message of the memory to which it is attached throughout the system. One part may hold the feeling of the spinning while another distributes it throughout the system, or one part may hold both jobs. When you find the parts who spin in order to distribute, you can substitute pleasant, warm, or courageous feelings for the destructive ones which are being spun.

In the meantime, if you are experiencing the spinning sensation, stand up straight, do not slump, focus outward, do not look down. Fight to hold onto the center of your body from the brain to your groin. Dig your feet into the ground. Drink a glass of water for grounding. The spinning episode is over. Fight for control. Focus on a large object in the room. Try to make it stand still. Focus on a medium sized one. Make it stop moving in your mind. Then a small one, then many small ones.

Try to walk to the bathroom. Count your steps. Stay away from the staircase. Eventually, the dizziness should stop. It pays to master the spinning because it could stop your process cold if you do not.

Give yourself permission to go beneath the spinning to the covered-over traumatic memory of being programmed.

This breakthrough can lead to an unravelling of memories that can set you on a path of listening to all your parts and coming to a most worthwhile freedom. It is one of the early steps to be mastered as fast as possible.

Sexual horrors

Wendy Hoffman

Survivors of mind control and ritual abuse usually become either promiscuous or averse to sexual expression and touch. They have suffered horrendous sexual abuse, more harrowing than most people would imagine. Their responses are inevitable. Anyone would react as they do.

Those pioneer therapists who treat survivors often try to help them bring back their sexuality in the hope that they will have a full life. Books have been written about reclaiming sexuality. Some of the earlier books address incest survivors. Incest is sufficient for ruining a life. Mind control victims also endure incest. Mind control victims grow up largely in electroshock chairs. Some are taken around the world to be programmed and tortured. Their minds are considered disposable software, their bodies toys for others' use. Perpetrators view them as servants or slaves with no inherent worth.

If you are a victim, keep in mind that you probably do not know the depths of your abuse, because you have been programmed to know nothing. If you are a therapist treating survivors, be aware that you do not know what your clients have been through. You may have a vague outline, but you will not know the chronic devastation and inconceivable abuses. The worst part of the sexual torture and training is well hidden in victims' internal systems and may be among the last portions of their history to emerge into consciousness. So, while the victim and his or her therapist(s) may strive to transform the victim into a normal functioning person or a focused sexual being limited to one partner, it might be useless because neither the victim nor the therapist knows what they are dealing with.

Sexual trainings take place in electroshock chairs. There, small—smaller than you can believe—children are masturbated. When their stirrings are achieved, programmers electroshock them—on their sexual parts. This is done for both boys and girls. Experts introduce children to premature sexual feelings, which are immediately coupled with physical pain. Children are sexually stimulated while viewing violent films or watching others tortured, to pair their sexual responses with violence. They are sexually stimulated while being placed next to dead bodies. They are forced to engage in sex with animals. They are forced to sexually abuse animals and other children, and may be sexually pleasured while they do it, to turn them into perpetrators. And, of course, they are forced to pleasure their handlers in whatever way those handlers want.

The combination of humiliation, violence, and physical pain creates confusion, then horror. Most children become divorced from their bodies. It will be a long, slow, circuitous route back. Take your time. Therapists—you cannot know. And if you are a bystander, support person, or witness, do not gawk.

Other child victims whom the leaders of these cults consider property are also used to stimulate the child victim in the chair. This is only one way perpetrators turn children against one another. At the end of these continuous sessions, the victims have lost their identities and function as created prostitutes, spies, tempters and temptresses, thieves, murderers, pornography players, and breeders.

What I am describing is official programming. The leaders never let programming go to waste. Cues such as the three of clubs and the queen of clubs are shown to the victims as they are tortured sexually. Victims then associate that card with the sexual torture and the behaviors they have to perform. In addition, as a small child is being prepared for a life of sexual slavery, the programmer will snap his fingers and point to a person in the room. Eventually the child learns to direct his or her sexual stirrings to that target pointed at.

Programming is un-American in that nothing goes to waste. The association of visual cues such as cards with the significance and memory of the programming mean that programmers and handlers can access and put into effect the programming at any moment of the victim's life. These sexual programs are sometimes turned on accidentally. Victims then have to deal with embarrassment and another kind of humiliation as well.

Some groups also make children copulate with animals. All groups favor penetration at an age considered too young by modern-world standards. Groups bring in mentally deficient males to rape ten- and eleven-year olds brutally and continuously. They drug these males so that they can hold erections. No one listens to these men when they do not want to hurt others and when they resist.

Victims sometimes do not understand why they have an aversion or addiction to touch and sex. Understanding some of the standardized training may help victims explain themselves to themselves and be more self-forgiving. A first step is always to bring abuses to light.

Survivors, though many do not realize it, live in stunned skin.

They have survived many invisible deaths.

To try to heal from the impossible, touch any innocuous place on your body. Notice whether the rest of you hops away. Do that until you can stay within yourself on that spot that you touched. Go on to other discrete spots.

Touch again. Do you associate touch with physical pain? Does some part of you shake as if in the after-vibrations of electroshock? Do you visualize many perpetrators? Gang rapes are common during and after programming sessions.

Do you associate touch with death? Orgies begin after the sacrifice(s) during rituals. Eventually survivors' crying in the present will most likely stop on its own, though it may take many years. Many survivors cry after orgasms in the present. That, too, might eventually cease.

This is the deep recovery work of a lifetime. You can decide whether to master it or not. It is your decision and no one else's. If you are in your twenties, thirties, or forties, your hormones may decide for you.

People can live without a sexual life. Or people can live with one. Sometimes things are ruined for good, and sometimes they are not.

The most important issue is to come back to your body gradually. Living within yourself is what is most important—living attached to yourself, owning yourself, belonging to yourself and having an aware mind. An aware mind is a solid single piece, and no longer fractioned.

Should you have a sexual body memory, pursue it, follow it to its end. Knowing what happened to you, what you endured, has to fill you with the self-esteem that has been stolen. You may come to love and cherish, honor and obey your own self.

Anger displacement training

Wendy Hoffman

Children's intense feelings are the seeds programmers work with. They take these emotions and direct them where it will profit the criminal group.

Programmers manipulate anger in children, starting almost at birth. They deliberately frustrate and enrage infants by taking away love, bottles, soft objects to cuddle. By the time their victims are toddlers, they are training them to kill. Given that they are creating an army of killers, they have to be able to control their victims' anger and direct it to their own enemies. Since they are the child's real enemies, it would be dangerous for them to leave anger intact and aimed at them. Depending on how fast the child develops, programmers wait until the children are about four to six years old to start teaching them not to be angry at their perpetrators but to direct that anger instead to this group's enemies. Their enemies include anyone who tries to help the child victims escape.

Here are some of the methods my family perpetrators used on me. Starting in 1948, when I was five, the programmers placed two archery targets with bulls-eyes on stands near the far wall in the basement. I had already achieved a good aim. The controllers taunted me and encouraged me to direct the frustration and anger I felt at my parents and sister onto those targets. Max, my main master-mind-programmer, instructed me to pull my anger from one target to the other one, while his younger brother, Abe, held a gun to my left temple and said, "Get it off that target and onto the other target or I'll pull this trigger." I had already endured "gun programming," which instructs complete obedience when a gun is held to you. When I was five to ten years old, I had to perform this transference of anger 100 times per session and when I was a teenager, 150 times per session. They strove for a spontaneous reflex I would perform without thinking. When I was a young teenager, the controllers laced three babies into seats and told me the babies would be killed if I did not transfer my anger correctly. I thought they were live babies, though possibly drugged. In addition, they gave me stimulant drugs that kept me in a riled-up mood but cooperative, the way the military drug soldiers in the known world.

Max and Abe knew I had transferred the anger when my eyes moved and I created another internal split. Particularly astute programmers can see when splits are created. As the training proceeded, I was forced to project my anger away from its original source and onto ten targets. Whatever I originally and rightly felt anger toward moved far away from my awareness. Anger became like boiling black smoke, beyond rage, not even human, demonic.

They wrapped my whole body in thick flesh-colored rubber like a space suit with a big opening around my back. My face and any bodily features did not show. I could feel the gun in my back and the taser blasts.

They had me walk to the first target and then suddenly pivot to the second or wherever they pointed. They shot at the spot I had just left, so that gun smoke always followed at my heels. They kept training me until my mind deflected automatically like a reflex. This became part of my training for killing politicians. All the internal kids had deflect-anger core training. The anger was held by a thousand child soldiers within me. Back at home, my grandmother shaved my scalp and told me that I had no identity.

With this training, they thought they could get me to do anything, and I could feel my brainwaves not holding a center and going every which way. The programmers told these parts whom to kill or blackmail or hurt. They had me not only walk, but crawl, walk backward, jump on both feet, walk on my toes, on my heels, hop, walk on my hands while they held my legs, roll on the floor, do leapfrog jumps, and do cartwheels, which I cannot do. They kept repeating the patterns with different movements to reinforce them.

Programmers put me in a coffin. Abe and Max pretended to put the coffin in my body, right where the spine ends, at my atlas. They pressed into my body at that location. They also banged my head to cause a concussion. Concussions make people passive and compliant and unable to think clearly. When I blacked out, the neighborhood cult-owned doctor would inject me and give me smelling salts to pull me out of it.

The men all pointed guns at me. I still wore that rubber suit when Uncle Abe said, "The old Wendy is dead; you are now a soldier, and all the soldiers stay in this coffin unless they're called out." He produced a sound pattern of knocks that the soldiers had to listen for. When the soldiers are out, everybody else has to go in the coffin. The coffins came in different sizes, always a tight fit. They also taught me visual symbols to provoke the transference of anger. Eventually, my mind could no longer hold the awareness of who had really caused the anger.

My family watched Apache dances, popular for decades starting in the 1930s, on the television in the living room. That was the trigger in ordinary life, but downstairs, starting when I was about five years old, in the lowest basement level with Max, and two uncles-in-law, I watched these dances while they kicked and masturbated me and gave these parts of me names.

Max told me that I was the woman in the dance and to put my anger in an empty can of Heinz vegetarian baked beans that he placed on the ground. (Mother served those beans a lot because we were not allowed to eat meat.)

I watched the show while they kicked me and tried to direct my anger to the can. Downstairs, they did not show the part of the dance where the woman abuses the man, but I saw that section upstairs in the living room. An uncle directed my anger to the can, then to large white dolls made of heavy white cloth and told me to be angry at this person and that person. The dolls were male and female with penises and pubic hair but no other features.

When they electroshocked me in the upstairs room with the black electroshock chair, I saw that they had placed the can in this room.

"You never saw this," my mind controller instructed. One of the uncles opened the window and my body became cold. "A layer of cold to seal in your memory."

At the end of this sequence, the uncle who kicked the hardest put me in a white laundry basket, covered me with a pink sheet and wheeled me home. He lifted me out and dumped me on the foyer floor of the apartment. Mother said, "You cannot leave her there." He dumped me on my bed. I would notice that laundry basket in the building's laundry room but would not have memories of the anger training. However, something in me resonated.

When I was an adult, my new programmers went back to this training, using similar methods. They pulled my hair and threw me around, as in Apache dances.

There has been significant discussion in recent decades about the innate differences and similarities between males and females. Displaced anger training gives glimpses of some differences. Starting at four or five years old, most male children took to anger more readily than the females. Girls took more readily to grief. Perpetrators use drugs to instill and enhance the feeling of anger. Some of the girls were overdosed because they did not get angry enough, and the controllers kept upping the drugs, always used in anger training (and probably military training).

How to make an assassin

Wendy Hoffman

One of the most dangerous and soul-wrenching mind control assignments is to be forced to become a murderer.

Little girls, and sometimes little boys, are trained to seduce, perform lap dances, drop pills in victims' drinks, and escape as their victims become drowsy, sick, or die, and to pull the trigger of guns. The same brain part does not perform the whole of this criminal act. A sequence of seven to ten parts, sometimes as many as fifteen, which are isolated from the rest of the brain, runs through these paces. During the childhood trainings, which start when the victim is a toddler, drugs and torture are used as well as a metronome to hypnotize and a stick pounding to accelerate the switches from one brain part to another. The switches have to be instantaneous and invisible. The programmers then seal or close the training. They use words, hand and foot signals, icons, or sounds to open the program on demand.

For assassination training with guns, the leaders train agile children to have excellent aim, first at archery ranges, then at shooting ranges. For their big job, they are trained to arrive at a destination, switch into another part, position themselves, switch, do a preparatory aim with their weapon, switch, watch for the signal from their handlers, switch, practice aim and reposition again, switch, obey their handlers' signal, switch, shoot, and finally switch into a part who knows nothing about what just happened. Assassins can also have their switches choreographed to songs in the assassin's head so that they do not need an external handler continually present when on a mission. The series of songs in the head (following a particular music album) may be externally triggered but then continue in a prescribed pattern internally. This programming can be disabled by an external person like a therapist speaking the lengths of songs on the album, followed by "If you've finished with the program, turn it off" (spoken in a particular tone of voice).

Assassins are equipped with suicide pills in case something goes wrong. Some assassins will be trained to stay put and be captured, others to run and be captured, others to escape. It depends on whether the leaders want to reuse this assassin. If the job is considered a particularly big one that involves, say, a charismatic political leader, sometimes a handler will accompany the assassin to the site, give him or her a signal such as a tap on the left shoulder, and even be present as the programmed assassin pulls the trigger. Handlers then disappear into the chaotic crowd. The trained assassin is often put in position to take the blame and is not really the one who murdered the target. Other killers shooting from other directions will have murdered the victim but they will disappear undetected and the known assassin will be discovered with a gun. He will shoot but his bullet will not be the one that killed. This duplicity is not usually discovered because these cult leaders have placed their own in the roles of agents investigating the crimes.

Most parts of the assassin's brain have no awareness that the body has just been to a public event and murdered a stranger. People designated as assassins are not usually given high positions in life. They are usually, but not always, kept as fringe citizens. Victims have other types of training for assassination roles, depending on the groups' preference. These are just a few examples.

The sections of victims' brains that are designated to be assassins are not allowed to be impulsive, but to just follow orders coolly and methodically. Nevertheless, some trained assassins snap out of that role and shoot the wrong person, often a handler who is at the scene, a relative, or someone they perceive to be particularly evil. The film *The Manchurian Candidate* depicts an assassin shooting his handler. And in my second memoir, *White Witch in a Black Robe*, I describe rotating my gun away from my assigned target, a good man, and onto the person at the table whom I considered particularly evil and conspiratorial.

Imprisoned assassins who say they do not remember killing anyone or shooting or owning a gun are probably telling the truth. The parts of their minds that hold the information have not come forward because their jailers do not know or do not use the codes to bring those parts forward. In the film *The Manchurian Candidate*, playing cards were the visual signal to bring forth the assassin-sequence of the protagonist. The cue could also be a song, melody, or body signal. In time, mind control often loses its power if not reinforced. To prevent this disintegration, jailed assassins may be reprogrammed while in prison.

Regular citizens in today's world are troubled by the assassinations and bombings taking place even in schools. Some of these might be to stir up chaos so that people will want a very controlling government. Trained slave-assassins and bombers are handed the weapons and ammunition needed for their jobs. Or there are stashes of weapons left for them in secret locations.

The leadership in perpetrator groups are accelerating the upheavals in the world, while the common man does not know what is going on and is afraid. The key to peace is to uncover the hidden rulers who are giving these instructions and the minor programmers who are training the future assassins. Right now, we are punishing the wrong people

Gang wars and the bandwagon

Wendy Hoffman

A much more benign form of victims' anger training than assassin training is when they are instructed to join an angry cult cause. One of the functions of some bits and pieces of the programmed mind is to disrupt non-cult activities that are designed to help survivors become free. For example, if a cult team leader is attacking a moderator on an on-line discussion board meant to support survivors, they will attack without thinking. For them, it is as if the whole world is a ritual site and they leap into the horrid festivities because that is what they have been tortured into doing. On communication boards for the professionals treating survivors, some of who are survivors themselves, we see the same sort of dynamics. People jumping on a cause, even a bad one, with compelling momentum.

When I assumed the position of moderator of an on-line communication board for survivors of mind control and ritual abuse, I had not thought I would run into great difficulties. My already published books had let people know that I am an advocate for victims of these horrendous abuses.

The previous moderator wanted to give up her role and start other endeavors. I had to abruptly take over, before the participants knew me. Just about immediately, attacks began. Fairly vicious attacks. Many of the participants on this well attended message board, I am sure, are lovely people. Some may not be, but the majority were most likely acting out of character. I was amazed at the animosity from otherwise fine people. Alison had a similar experience when she did two webinars for a survivor organization. She presented sound material that was going to be in her books. Almost as soon as she began speaking, people began to interrupt, saying, "That's triggering," or "That triggered me," or "That's so upsetting." She was unable to get through her prepared material.

The programs behind this are called "gang war" and "hop on the bandwagon." I went into my own past to find out how it works. I am sure there are many varieties and innovations.

1940s: First I found programming that happened when I was five or six. It took place in the programming center underneath the apartment building my family lived in. The perpetrators were my parents, aunts, and uncles. The main command said, "There will be an infringement of justice. Everyone has to get angry." Each infringement was ridiculous.

To initiate the training, my mother was told to object to red traffic lights when she wanted to cross the street. Why should she have to wait for a light? The other females in this basement said, "It's not fair, you are unjust, you are a tyrant." I had to join in. I said something like "The red light regulates traffic and is necessary so that everyone, cars and people, do not go together." That was before the program took effect.

The master programmer whipped me. He threatened me, saying he would take away all my toys, that I would never be allowed outside again, that I had to follow my leaders or I would not be allowed to live. The whipping on my back and legs was hard. The seeds of this programming were planted.

My mother was directed to say something like "Rah." The word meant nothing. Then the aunts said it. I had to say "Rah," then other vague sounds. Then we graduated to expressions such as "It's not fair." And so on. If I did not participate by joining this gang, the programmer strangled me, almost to death. Gasping, I was placed on the electroshock chair. He tightened the head vise and said: "You will always follow your leader. You will always join your team. You will always protest when they protest injustice." Injustice is the key falseword. Drugs made me more compliant.

I received other trainings with deeper threats as I aged. In my twenties, at a government facility, the program was called "Hop on the band wagon:" Programmers showed me a picture of a small bus. I could also see a real one that was in an area below. The programmer instructed, "When someone indicates anger because of an injustice, you hop on the bandwagon. It doesn't matter whether you agree. It is your job to back your team. You express the anger while your team leader is quiet. Sometimes you will not know who your team leader is. You are the voice. You are the voice for justice. Holler for your compatriots. This is a government command."

A little later, I was in a very sophisticated black chair with a head vise with a huge helmet attached. The male programmer spoke as female assistants in white uniforms surrounded him.

"You are an ant in a giant colony. You never act on your own. When your team leader shows distress, you listen carefully. When he lifts the pinky and index fingers of his left hand, you start yelling at the source of his distress. You do the noisy, dirty work. He is then silent and satisfied. It's as if he is getting a blow-job. You simply make noise and make your team leader look innocent."

In the same decade, the infamous Dr. Cameron at McGill Hospital programmed me after I did not follow instructions to assassinate one of their enemies. This programming took place when I was disobedient.

Dr. Cameron: "You always follow your leader. If he points, you do. You jumped on the wrong bus. You should be executed. You have been trained and you did everything wrong. The leader points, you shoot. You are the voice, not a wild fire."

He continued: "You had a team there and you did not hop on the bandwagon. You wanted your own way and you made trouble. Trouble. I'll put you in the ovens. You Jewish-bitch-queen." Saliva dripped from his distorted mouth.

Sometimes, in the 1980s, my front person was aware when I hopped on the bandwagon even though the fight had no personal benefit for me. But the compulsion was great and I could not stop myself. My then handler would indicate something he was upset about and leave the protest to me.

The leaders of these attacks are usually more sedate than those programmed to join the bandwagon. Sometimes the leaders are so behind the scenes that observers do not even know of their existences.

They control their noisy followers by pushing invisible program buttons. The leaders may be "conscious." They are usually cult-loyal and dangerous. It is easy to blame the pushy followers, but the real disruptions come from the sometimes invisible leaders. As a co-moderator of one of the discussion boards for survivors, I sometimes could not tell the difference between the leaders who initiated the attacks and all the followers who picked up the energy and ran with it.

If you are a survivor, ask yourself whether you ever jump into fights or arguments even though you have nothing to gain.

Do you feel compelled to back up someone you might think of as a friend but who may really be your handler or team leader, even when this leader is working against you?

The beginning step in breaking this training is to become aware of the compulsion to enter conflicts that do not serve your purposes. You, too, can step away from fighting and attacking in order to receive rather than sabotage the help you need.

If you are a therapist and are seeing gang wars and bandwagon hopping in your professional networks, look at who is involved. They may be the cult moles (plants) you need to identify.

In love with death

Wendy Hoffman

Satanic cults create a culture of death and dying. Death becomes attached to survivors' skin. Leaders like to join death and birth. Sacrifices of infants, children, and adults often take place during rituals that include births. Or a pregnant victim gives birth and is simultaneously murdered. I have seen that happen. She was told that if she did not scream, the murderers would not also kill her newborn. The child lived.

Survivors, possibly all survivors, have witnessed murders. War soldiers, genocide survivors, ghetto gang members have also seen multiple murders. Soldiers have witnessed massive deaths within a relatively short time, several months to a decade. War in ordinary life is usually not hidden. At least the people who endure it know it is happening. In criminal mind control cults, there is ordinary life and the hidden secret life of death rituals and assignments. Only parts of the person know about the underside life, and most of society does not know and would not believe it. Knowledge of its existence is probably more prevalent now than ever before. Mind control survivors live with death or the threat of death either their whole lives or until they are able to break away from the criminal groups and remain safe.

Witnessing death, even more than the other abuses, eliminates the possibility of a childhood. Satanic cult children are like William Blake's chimney sweeps, thrust into an adult world of violence and grime that erases the possibility of innocence. Their untimely exposure to sex seals the lid.

Leaders and programmers weave death into all their mind control programs. For example, when telling someone what not to do, they like to say "upon penalty of death".

After the murder of the one friend allowed, death becomes associated with inconsolable loss and guilt, all pre-planned. Some survivors are left with huge guilt feelings. No matter what happens, they feel guilty. Others become so numb that they cannot see when they do anything wrong. Feelings of tragic loss follow survivors everywhere.

Some of the "deaths" they witnessed did not actually happen. Children were tricked and the deaths were falsified. But child survivors in particular think they happened, so the effects are just as damaging and lasting as if the murders were real. Programmers also like to create the illusion of an after-life. They use magic tricks to make children believe they are seeing souls emerging from dead bodies to be trapped and caught. They tell the children that internal librarians, or managers, are placing the souls in boxes and that the boxes are being placed inside the child victims. Or they say file cabinets or caskets, vaults, caves, or some other kind of container. Children will feel that the dead live within them. They are afraid of some of the spirits but do not know how to get away from them. They have the mistaken impression that whole graveyards exist within them as well as ancient souls and spirits from other times and lands. Moreover, children are tricked into thinking they can catch souls with their fingers and hands. Trainers have drugged children, taught them to separate yolks from the white portion of eggs and tell them that they are catching souls. Lighting effects at rituals emulate spirits rising from the ritual site to "Lucifer's heavens."

Survivors are sometimes aware of the dead as they live their lives. The murdered dead whom the survivor loved can stay with that person in life. Some cherished dead friends protect and comfort them. The sense of their presence has a strong impact on survivors and keeps them going. Survivors may over-know death, but they also know the depth of love.

Their exterior world is filled with exposure to death; they believe their insides are filled with representations of death, and their programming is filled with death. Once your mind is taken away from you and you do not have free will, you become like the dead. Robots are not alive. Automatons live trance-like existences.

In addition, almost every survivor is loaded with suicidal ideation. Parents teach their small children how to kill themselves. These parents are told that if they do not, their children will be skinned and killed, so they teach their children to slit their wrists, jump out of windows, overdose on their parents' obviously placed medications, to name just a few ways. Simultaneously, programs exist for homicidal acts. Children are carefully taught how to murder and how to dissect corpses. The training starts with fish, birds, and small animals as targets and progresses to humans.

Even as some cult children are born to be murdered early in their lives, some are born who are not allowed to be killed until later in their adulthood or old age. It is typical of the arrogance of this kind of satanism to assign expiration dates to some of their victims. Those not allowed to be murdered until late in their lives will be born into positions these cults consider higher and more important than average. If these individuals are not obedient, they will be tortured but not killed. They may have long lives of torture until they either break free or are finally murdered. They may be considered even more unfortunate then the "expendables" murdered early in life. I am one of these unfortunates.

The only way to get away from all this death and make-believe death and killing and the compulsion to kill yourself is to undo the programming. Run away from your perpetrators, do not tell them where you are, and, in safety and calm, start unravelling their commands, one program at a time, one mandate after another, until you are free and clear of all the programs they imposed on your brain. It is the only way to step away from a religion of death and dying and into life. Wash the residue of death off your skin. Let your pores breathe in life. Leave death's stench behind.

Politicians' use of victims

Wendy Hoffman

Hordes of victims from multi-generational cult families are trained from birth onward to service politicians and people scheduled to be in power eventually, including world leaders. They serve as sexual slaves, memorizers, and messengers. The sexual slaves perform in private or in groups, on yachts and in homes, including official palaces and government-assigned homes. They often have permanent genital markings that indicate to perpetrators that they have been molded for this heinous role. They will service and not talk and not remember. Meanwhile the political figures go off satisfied, self-righteous, not endangered, revered, and scot-free.

Some of these children are subjugated young and taught to use their brains as a camera or tape recorder. Click, they can record words. Click, click—they can record documents. They then travel to the next politicians or businesspeople and deliver the information in words. Some function as mules who deliver elite drugs and/or messages and instructions in writing. Programmers construct them to dissociate this knowledge. But survivors are beginning to leak. Some have memories of being trained for, and performing, these roles, including those of political assassins. Some have written about this aspect of their lives. I have. Even within those survivors who do not yet have conscious memories, an earthquake rumbles and sways. When political primaries and campaigns are in full flood, memories threaten to erupt. Many victims do not understand why they feel so triggered day after day. The faces on television and the internet do not stop. Somewhere deep inside, the victims are aware that they know these people. Some cannot find words to express their impressions. Others' clarity is sharp. They overcome the "do not know, do not tell" commands. They recognize the hand signals given at significant times—hand signals reminding them not to tell. In a certain context, such a signal could be translated into a command not to say anything bad about a certain candidate.

So, survivors know or are beginning to know. But whom can they tell? People who have not been mind-controlled and programmed through torture do not want to know. The vitriol the 2016 candidates inspired was astounding. Friendships ended. Neighbors stopped talking to one another. Huge signs promoting one or another candidate appal people. In rural communities, stores exhibit such signs. Some customers will no longer enter them.

Only the politically visible perpetrators, diminished survivors, and some of their therapists and support people know what is going on. Perpetrators do not want to talk and survivors are not allowed to, even if they remember what happened. On professional discussion online sites, therapists are not allowed to say what they know about politicians. On survivor sites, survivors are not permitted to name names. The world from every angle conspires to keep the *status quo* in place and survivors muzzled. Ordinary people do not need hand signals instilled through torture and mind control not to be aware. Even survivors who have achieved freedom and remember the themes of their lives find they have to sit on their truths. All sides buffet them.

The perpetrator groups work hard to disguise perpetrators' identities to victims. Some confused survivors have spoken out identifying the wrong people as perpetrators, because of their programming. Others might be deliberately misidentifying good people. But credible survivors who have reached a good degree of health are giving consistent information.

Which is worse: continuing to be mind-controlled or being the little boy who cried "The emperor has no clothes" and being punished with ongoing torture for speaking out? This is not a fairy tale and so far has not had a happy ending. Survivors end up alienated either by mind control or knowledge. We still live in the aftermath of Stalin. As a mob, we cheer the wrong people.

Twenty-first century Nazis

Wendy Hoffman

It is easy to underestimate the influence and power of today's Nazism. Some of its less educated members do blatantly Nazi acts, but the more educated ones, with power and position in society, hold their meetings and rituals in secret and use mind control procedures. Only recently have photographs emerged of a seven-year-old Queen Elizabeth and members of the British royal family doing Nazi salutes. Joe Kennedy's affiliation with Nazi leaders cost him his office decades ago.

What does Nazism express that appeals to both the poor and the very rich? It represents power and annihilation—destruction.

My legal father, the one who raised me, who married my mother in ordinary life and pretended to be my biological father, came from a Nazi family. My mother's side of the family was Illuminati and wanted their group to rule the world as did my father's side.

My son's wedding was engineered by cult people, and it never occurred to me that my son's wife came from a Nazi family. They were nominal Christians who lived in Hillary Clinton's borough. I never saw them lynch blacks. But perhaps that's a portrait of many Nazis.

Why would the cults want to marry Nazis to Jewish people? Modern-day Nazism is different from Hitler's in some ways. Hitler attempted to exterminate all Jewish people and leave not a trace. Modern-day Nazis want to take those they hate and convert them to their way of thinking. Historic Nazis tried to rid their communities of foreigners and anyone they deemed socially unacceptable. They eliminated Jews, whereas the modern-day Nazis intermarry with Jewish people as a way of eliminating Judaism.

Right before the wedding, my son's wife's family did a ritual that I describe in *The Enslaved Queen* and in which my son and I were being abused. The chanters made negative comments about our being Jewish but I did not put it all together. Later, I remembered a programming session that same pre-wedding night that preceded the remembered ritual. Hoodlums abducted me from the hotel and took me by car to an apartment building where all the mailboxes had false Arab names. They all seemed Arab. A woman in a burkha was on the main floor, as my daughter-in-law, her sister, and her mother held guns pressed into my back and walked me up the steps. There were humiliations for me and my son. The perpetrators wanted to make us think we were dogs, then came the standard tortures.

When I told Alison about this, she asked whether I could see the torturers' hands and what color they were. I saw hands whose skin color was lighter than mine, one with red hairs. Horrible things were said about the Jewish people as spit flew from their mouths. After the torture, the programmers showed me photos such as mug-shots of the Boston bombers and other mind-controlled Arab terrorists. They commanded me to believe my abusers at this time were Muslim terrorists and not the white supremacist Nazis they really were. At the end, the apparently Arab woman on the first floor cleaned me up. She was the token to reinforce the idea that I had fallen into Arabs' hands.

The mechanics of this memory give one example of how hidden the Nazi groups are in today's world—not the thugs who roam the streets, but the people who hold respectable positions in the world and even world leaders. It also tells of the enhanced tricks they will use to disguise their identities and pin their misdeeds on other groups.

The frequency of programming

Wendy Hoffman

When survivors start their memory process, they pull out from their tightly closed minds a memory here, a memory there. These often turn out not to be the worst memories, but they are often representative of some of the major themes in their usurped lives. Years go by, and survivors working on associating or bringing to consciousness what their lives have been can fill large sacks with personal retrieved information. Eventually, they see themselves in black chairs and their understanding of programming for mind control begins. The black chair, indicating electroshock, is often one of the most telling keys to knowledge. Their perpetrator list grows. The relatives survivors thought they had loving relationships with may be the last ones recalled, as well as the well-known and idealized political, religious, social, athletic, and artist personalities. The private and world arenas collapse for them then.

These realizations are agonizing, but the big realization is yet to come. Until now, the awareness has been of an event here and there. Suddenly, those barriers fall away. As they crumble, a grid-like life comes into focus. It was not an occasion here and there that covered a programming session where the mind was erased and a new one installed. It was not only something that happened when the victim was three, six, eighteen, twenty-four, and so on. It was constant! The shock of this realization makes one's earth tremble.

Recovery can be divided into before this realization and after this realization.

Before, you thought nice things also occurred in your tarnished life. You thought you went on that road trip with your father because he loved you. It was your special time together. If you are a parent, you thought your adult child visited you because he cared about you and missed you. All these events stacked up in your life, but now you realize that they were covers or excuses to get you to a location where your perpetrators would administer additional programming and mind control.

The nice moments of your life flew out the window. It was all a lie. A horribly gigantic lie.

If you get away from your controllers, in time your mind control will lessen and perhaps become ineffective. But if your controllers know where you are and have access to you, they will resurrect the diminishing programming and refresh your mind control. That is one of the reasons it is essential not to report your intentions or preference for freedom or your location if you have run away.

With the illusion of having the nice moments of your life gone, then what do you have?

Reality, truth, and, for the first time, belonging to yourself at last. Is that enough? It will have to be.

There is more. They decided on the work you would do both in the secret organizations you were born into and in ordinary, normal life. They decided whom you would marry and where you would live. You could not even buy a house without their permission—or even a dog. You could not give your children lessons without their say-so. You could not send your children to a specialized school without their permission.

They fabricated every stitch of your life.

The commanders even decide which facial expressions victims will wear. My ex-ordinary-life husband assumed a sweet expression to cover his crude meanness. My ex-cult-husband learned after years of practice to make his face devoid of feeling. Mind-controlled assassins are taught to exhibit smug, self-satisfied facial expressions when they are caught. These looks infuriate the general public. The Boston bombers and the Orlando terrorist had the same kind of taught expressions on their self-satisfied faces. Assassins sometimes appear genuinely confused, since they do not know that they are stooges.

It seems that the first step in freedom is grief. They stole everything.

You are left now with your present and future. No matter how old you are when you become aware, seize every moment of what is left now. Hold tight to yourself, the self that belongs to you alone. Hold tight. You worked so very hard to get here. Despite the heart-breaking grief, you are yours alone now. No one owns you. Your mind can be in one piece.

As I neared the end of my processes of associating my lost past, I became tired and weary. *How much more will I have to go through?* I sighed. Then came the awareness that the programming and control were constant and that I had no free will during my life. I cannot process millions of programming sessions both in and out of their chambers. I will skim over and search for anything new or irregular in those myriad memories. I will investigate deeply the ones that contain a deviation or difference. The rest will have to wash away as a group. Often, there are not that many years left to live. I want to put my energy into life, since for me life is what is new and different.

I do not know whether survivors ever reach the end of associating the imposed dissociation. It is, however, important to believe that there will be an end to these horrendous memories and disillusionment about people and society.

Whether or not you ever get to the pivotal memories, you have the right to define yourself and not be made into a non-human being, a machine following orders.

Conscious and unconscious perpetrators

Alison Miller

The first person to tell me about "going conscious" was the late Stella Katz, the programmer whose unimaginable piece on Kaballah programming I published in *Healing the Unimaginable*. Stella was in the process of systematically working through her own training memories during the day when her husband was at work and her children were at school. Being a cult programmer, she knew how her memories were stored internally, and she knew that she must put together every part of a memory in order to destroy the program it had created. Stella described herself as having "a case of galloping integration." She was thirty-nine years old, and that was the age at which she had been supposed to "go conscious"—that is, to have the parts who lived her everyday life join with the parts who were loyal to the cult who had trained her, while the hurt child parts were to be hidden under a barrier where they would not be found. She was using the "go conscious" program for her own ends, following the laid out path which those who trained her had intended, removing the barriers within her inner structure one section at a time, but defeating the cult's purpose by including the hurt child parts in the joining. The program was supposed to work gradually, integrating one internal group at a time. She worked hard on it every day, because, she said, if even one child part remains within the system, the present-day programmers can access that part to split it once more.

I do not know the entire method by which a person becomes conscious, whether it is entirely an internal process led by a few hidden insiders who change the structure to make parts share their knowledge, or whether it requires an external person to set it off. That is because "conscious" members of these groups do not generally go for therapy. I only know what I have learned from Stella and Wendy, both of whom refused the demand to become "conscious."

If a person goes conscious, he or she becomes a conscious perpetrator, fully identified with the goals of the group, rewarded with status and power and freedom from being tortured. Only people of high status in the perpetrator groups are given the option of going conscious, and they are presented with this decision at designated ages in adulthood. Wendy was repeatedly asked to go conscious, and she repeatedly refused. She did not want to lose her soul. She was supposed to take part in a ceremony to become "conscious" at the 1982 Feast of the Beast ritual, when she would have been thirty-nine, like Stella. Prior to that ritual she would probably have undergone gradual changes in her internal structure and personality system. Her decision to refuse this offer meant a life of pursuit and torture rather than comfortable wealth and authority.

Many people who are not "conscious" are still working for the groups in one way or another. Wendy, for example, was working as a therapist and expected to use methods taught to her to close down those clients who had lived through these abuses. She wrote about this in *The Enslaved Queen*. Survivors of mind control and ritual abuse are sent to conferences or email discussion lists with parts of them instructed to use hand signals or code words to trigger programming in other vulnerable survivors. They are generally unaware that they are doing this. But other members of the conferences or lists are "conscious," and are aware of what they are triggering and why. They may be given jobs such as "matriarch," offering apparent comfort and support and gathering victims to follow their hidden instructions. Or they may be programmers, taking people into hotel rooms or out in vans during conferences and reinforcing those people's programming through torture.

I do not know whether it is possible to undo "going conscious." Perhaps if someone had accepted this without fully understanding its implications, then recognized that he or she had hidden hurt child parts, such a person could find where the parts were hidden and work through their pain. This is close to what Stella chose to do, when she allowed the program to work gradually but subverted its purpose to achieve full integration.

Persons who have become "conscious" are given positions where they are responsible for advancing the agenda of the perpetrator groups. Wendy notes that the conscious people who have their inner children repressed can still rage and have tantrums. They appear hollow, but also as if they are drowning. Many children grow up surrounded by "conscious" adults. The conscious are like the dead, and the ones who resist or are not considered stable enough or elevated enough in these criminal groups are sometimes driven insane. Those members who are given high political office or important positions in society are inevitably people who have gone conscious and over whom the rulers have complete control.

Things I wish I did not know

Alison Miller

Have you ever wondered why mind control and ritual abuse survivors all over the world report the same phenomena? As I wrote "Fifty lies they may have told you" in around 2014, I was reasonably sure that survivors in Germany, Australia, and South Africa would recognize some of the same lies that survivors in Canada and the USA have reported to me and to their therapists. The Extreme Abuse Survey (https://eassurvey.wordpress.com/extreme-abuse-survey-final-results/) asked about particular reported abuses, and found many to be common to survivors all over the world. Why are they common? Because perpetrator groups collaborate and teach one another techniques of torturing children, splitting the infant mind, and training mind-controlled victims.

It is *organized crime*. It is *psychologically sophisticated organized crime*. What else should we call it? Like the Mafia, it runs in families; people are born into it. And, as in the Mafia, those born into the families are expected to continue the family tradition of crime. I wish I did not know that. I wish I did not know so many people who, through no fault of their own, were born into it, and have endured lifelong torture, including child prostitution and pornography. I wish dogs, which I love, were not used as sacrifices. I wish children were not taught to rape and kill and then told they are evil and "possessed." When I worked with my first survivors, I thought there were a number of smaller groups in different locations who did roughly similar things. I did not realize the extent of the national and international organization of these groups. I have learned more about this from Wendy, because she was unlucky enough to be placed at the highest level within the international organization of some of the major groups. I wish I had not learned this. I wish I had not learned that politicians are involved, including world leaders. I wish I had not learned that some of my favorite musicians and film stars may have been involved, that the groups have a hand in deciding who rises to stardom.

I wish I had not learned recently that some people who purport to help survivors, including some well-known therapists, religious leaders, and leaders of non-profit groups, are actually members of perpetrator groups with jobs such as spreading disinformation or gathering and silencing survivors who had escaped. I wish that Christianity and Judaism and perhaps other religions had not been corrupted and misused by perpetrators. I wish that various schools of therapy had not been corrupted and misused by perpetrators. I wish that therapists were not teaching self-help techniques which are actually program triggers, sometimes in complete unawareness.

I wish I did not know these things. I wish I did not constantly walk a tightrope between naïvely trusting those who do not deserve my trust and fearfully suspecting everyone who may be trying to do good but do not understand the situation.

I wish I lived in the world my siblings live in, where they are appalled by some recent political events but are happy to spend their time gardening or travelling as tourists and playing golf, where law enforcement catches the perpetrators, where the biggest enemies are old age and cancer. I wish I lived in the world I lived in when I was young, where children played on the street and (as far as I knew) the neighbors looked after them safely. I wish I lived in the world I thought I lived in as a young adult, where God looked after those who tried to live good lives, and we could trust Him not to send us more than we could bear.

Survivors bear the unbearable through dissociation, segmentation of their brains into many parts. But this dissociation is exploited by abusers to control those brains, piece by piece. They struggle when they become aware of what they have gone through and might still be going through. Therapists, kind spouses, and support people struggle with the knowledge of such unbearable things. We have to revise our worldviews, and this is a painful but necessary process.

I wish I did not know all this. But people closed their eyes when Hitler was sending people to concentration camps to be killed. People in the "developed" countries close their eyes when genocides happen in the "less developed" countries. The UN would not send enough troops to save Rwanda, and would not intervene in Syria. The leaders of western "democracies" frame refugees as illegal immigrants and invaders of their people's safety and security, so that very few people recognize that these unfortunate people could be us.

We cannot close our eyes to these known abuses.

I have chosen not to close my eyes to mind control and ritual abuse. Even though I wish I did not know.

SECTION V
SAFETY

The "angel" of suicide

Wendy Hoffman

A mind-controlled slave cannot live making his or her own decisions. If you are a child learning to ride a bicycle, first you learn to operate the brakes. Then you will not crash into pedestrians and cars. If you are a child growing up within a criminal, high level mind-control cult, one of your first lessons is how to commit suicide. Then your controllers can eliminate you if you spring a leak, know too much, or are more rebellious than they can handle. Or if they need a dead person to take the blame for what they themselves do.

People will not want to kill themselves if they know that their death will be both painful and needless. Therefore, handlers fool the victim children into believing that death will lead them into a peaceful paradise. The children suffer so in every way that they yearn for some peace. Mostly, cult children experience inflicted pain, so the possibility of comfort attracts and excites them.

Controllers deliver an apparent angel to lead the way into this much desired fake paradise, which is, in reality, only a brutal death. In the crib, before the infant knows speech, handlers show images of the angel as they stroke, soothe, drug, and feed the famished baby. They use slide projectors, film, and computers to project the fake angel's movement around and across the room. Before babies have taken their first steps, they know this angel as a frequent companion. They associate its presence with comfort and freedom from pain, plus the angel looks beautiful, like a Renaissance painting. Babies never suspect duplicity. They do not have that concept.

Handlers use words as babies mature. "Follow the angel of mercy [or the angel of the sunset—by now, there must be many other words for this trick] and you will be well."

As babies become small children, programmers introduce triggers or cues that the children will eventually associate with the message and image of the angel. First, they torture the child, then drug the child, then show the child the angel. The angel becomes associated with the means of relief. They want the child to follow the angel wherever it leads. One survivor reported walking the Kaballah pathways in a cult training center, entering many rooms filled with torture and illusions such as puppets simulating demons. In the last room at the end of each pathway was a woman dressed up as the angel, who drugged the child and soothed her into sleep. At the end of my outdoor pathways, when I was a toddler and small child, when the terror and pain ended, there was often an image of the angel or a human dressed like this angel. The angel became associated with the end of torment.

A playing card such as the eight of spades, a letter in a foreign language, a musical or natural sound, or a tarot card picture is sufficient to invoke the image of this deceptive angel and its inherent message—"Follow me into death."

These trespasses are introduced in infancy. The victim grows to understand their meanings.

Starting right after toddlerhood, trainers, who are often parents and grandparents, teach children how to kill themselves. Each group will have a preferred method—jumping off a bridge or out of a window, drowning, slitting wrists, overdosing on an adult's pills. As victims grow older, handlers and other controllers will tell the person of all the bad things he or she has done and increase feelings of guilt and shame to an intolerable level. People might want to die just to get away from these intense feelings. Ironically, the victims might not have even performed many of the acts the controllers make them feel guilty about. All programming is based on deceptions.

Moreover, life as a mind-controlled slave is so painful, disturbing, and fruitless that death at times could seem like a blessing, but this kind of death is not. It is only the fulfillment of one's life as a slave and does not help you become the person you really are. Undoing this programming and attempting freedom are how survivors can redeem their, until now, unfortunate lives. Helping other survivors may add something to their lives as well.

Throughout life, slaves are drilled about when to kill themselves. The training is continuous. If a victim ever disobeys, if controllers ever give that person the signal, if he or she would ever reveal secret information, then controllers will want that person to kill themselves for the benefit of the group's security. Eventually, if the adult victim misbehaves or if the leaders just need a stooge, this program, already entrenched in the victim, will be activated.

This programming is enforced and re-enforced, which does not mean it cannot be broken. Once people understand the lies and manipulations, the programming dissolves, sometimes immediately and totally. The internal adults can help the inner children understand how they were fooled and lied to.

If you have survived these kinds of abuses and see an image of this sort of angel, know that it will only lead you to a bad kind of death. Try to unravel the programming that deceives you into thinking that this image or the symbol that evokes this association will in any way benefit you. Find the parts who hold this programming. Remember to go back to the earliest memories from the crib and include those.

You have a choice—to do what your handlers have trained you to do or to live the rest of your valuable life in your own way.

To die or not to die

Wendy Hoffman

I have always known from the depths of my being that I did not want to be alive. Who would want to be alive with a family like mine? Or some cult role like mine? I had eight children and I do not see a single one; neither do I know whether six of them are alive. I could pass five of them on the street and not know it. And the torture and denigration—unbearable. I am not writing this to complain. I am writing so that you will understand why I did not want to live. I only wanted to live for one year of my life, when my friend Daniel was alive and loved me.

So I wonder over and over why I remained alive. Was it fate or divine intervention? I did make some suicide attempts but they were not successful. I wondered about still being alive throughout all the years of my conscious recovery, but it was only this year, when I am seventy-two and pretty much integrated, that with Alison's help I remembered a do-not-die program.

On the one hand, my mother was teaching me to make "trees" along my arms and wrists with my father's razor blade. She seemed to take a special glee in teaching me to die. She also taught me to hold my head down in the bathtub.

At the same time, my biological father was teaching me to follow the Angel of Mercy to wherever it led—which would be to death.

So it was clear that my immediate family wanted me to know how to slit my wrists, drown, jump off bridges and roofs and crash.

Then why did they teach me simultaneously not to die?

The do not-die programming may have begun even before the suicidal programming.

On the roof of the apartment building where I grew up, my family strapped a harness around me. The harness had a very long leash attached. The programmer projected an image of this giant Angel of Mercy onto the sky. They told me at three years old, four years old, five and up to seven years old, to go to the edge of the roof. The Angel of Mercy lured me to the ridge, then blocked the other side of the ledge. It appeared that the angel blocked me, but the projectionist was really projecting the Angel's image between me and the sky. "Go back," the family all screamed together and tugged my harness backwards. I would have been happy to jump because I was already disillusioned with life, but they would not let me. "Daniel wants you alive." "You have to live." Over and over they led me to the ledge and then stopped the jump with the tug on the harness and their words.

Alison Miller describes similar trainings her clients received in her book, *Healing the Unimaginable* (2011, p. 188). Her clients were taught about hell in their cults and told that is where they would go if they killed themselves.

It is mind-boggling to be programmed in contradictory ways. I think most children growing up in the severely abusive and no-love atmosphere of generational mind-control cults would prefer death. But then they also have training to stay alive at all costs. This intentional mixing up of the mind and pulling it in opposite directions at once is typical of the insidious nature of organized, criminal mind control.

Once I discovered do-not-die programming, I felt disappointed. It was not divine intervention or fate. Once again, it was just mind control. I could not even choose whether to live or die.

Now that I am old and alive, I do not want to die. I want to expose these abuses, heal completely and help others heal. My programmers would not let me die. I will be so public, they will be sorry.

I understand the do-not-die programming. It takes effort, manpower, and money to mass produce automatons. They do not want all that work wasted. But if they are not going to let you die, why all the specific suicidal training? Is it to destroy self-esteem? Is it to give us the message that not only are we not loved and wanted, we also do not deserve to be alive?

One of the most painful lessons for Holocaust survivors was that many of the population wanted them exterminated, their whole race wiped off the earth. Perhaps the suicidal training for cult victims teaches them wrongly that they are considered similarly worthless and undesirable.

Those of us who have survived can show the world how resilient and worthy we are.

This dual and simultaneous programming of kill yourself/do-not-die affects the brain gravely. The parts inside who want to kill themselves and the parts who cannot are unable to coexist. This inability to coexist can create thicker and greater barriers. If a suicide program is acted on, its opposite will appear to wipe it out. That is not co-existence. It is dominance and eradication. It is dissociation that makes both "die" and "do not die" be present within the same person, without awareness of each other.

Programmed suicide and therapists

Alison Miller

Most therapists have received at least basic training in how to assess whether a client is suicidal, and how high the risk. They have also been instructed to take all suicide threats seriously, and to provide immediate service and possible hospitalization to clients with specific suicide plans or other risk factors.

All survivors of mind control and ritual abuse have suicide training. They also have "Do not die" training, as described in Wendy's previous essay. (The pairing of Die and Do not Die programming is typical of mind control. There is also Sleep–Do not Sleep and Run–Do not Run training.) Back to suicide: The perpetrator groups put a lot of time and money into training their mind-controlled victims, and they do not want them just escaping via death. I remember one client who detailed how she was taught exactly how many pills to take—one less than the amount that was potentially lethal.

At the same time, the suicide programming is very useful to the groups. If a survivor is working hard to get free, and the group cannot get hold of her, the perpetrators can trigger her suicide programming through a hand signal, and her mental health professionals will be obliged to hospitalize her, delivering her into the hands of the perpetrators on the hospital staff. If a survivor is remembering and telling about important known crimes, and is not very important to the group, the group might decide she is better off dead. It will help if she has made previous unsuccessful suicide attempts. That will make sure she has achieved the "Borderline" diagnosis, and has inconvenienced the care system sufficiently that they will just sigh when she eventually dies of apparent suicide. It will not even occur to her psychiatrist that it was actually murder. Two of my early clients who survived told me that the cult had broken into their apartments and forced all their pills down their throats in an attempt at murder disguised as suicide. Another one died (see Chapter One of *Healing the Unimaginable* (2011)), and her long history of suicide attempts came in useful to the perpetrators.

The Extreme Abuse Survey (see References section) discovered that mind control and ritual abuse survivors made many more suicide attempts than other extreme abuse survivors, but had no more successful suicides. So, therapists treating survivors need to be aware of the programming for unsuccessful suicide attempts and the "do not die" programming, as well as programming for successful suicide in cases in which the perpetrator group has decided the survivor is of no further use to them and might pose a risk. We need our own criteria for deciding whether a survivor client is a genuine suicide risk (on the basis of how much threat he or she poses to the perpetrator group), and if we believe a client is at genuine risk, we need to regard hospitalization as a last resort choice, unless we are 100% sure that our local hospital is not infiltrated by the perpetrator group. In my early years of working with survivors, I discovered that our local mental hospital was thoroughly infiltrated. The cult van made a regular stop at the front door during the dinner hour, to pick up survivors who came out "for a smoke," and reprogram them. I do not believe this is unusual.

Current contact

Wendy Hoffman

I have heard therapists refer to ongoing involvement with a perpetrator group as "current contact." That term implies agreement. It does not quite capture the situation. Cult members break into your home, terrorize and torture you, or they grab you off the street and take you somewhere to mind-control you, or they program you to appear at a designated place and time where they will do the same. This last option might be the worst because you have become even more the unwitting victim. None of these scenes imply consent.

Shall we call it, then, current abduction? Even in the third option, your mind has been abducted through formal mind control.

There are two reasons for current abduction: (1) your actions or words have indicated that you desire freedom and, therefore, have to be crushed and packaged in torture immediately. Or (2) the group that claims you does maintenance work and schedules mind-control sessions and rituals regularly throughout the year, in addition to formal holidays. You are programmed to attend, and might be punished severely if you do not.

Concerning break-ins for the purpose of stopping a quest for freedom, it is rarely one person who will break into your home. The group will have one programmer, and one or more people trained to administer torture to your body and possibly that of your pet(s). Since they will not have an electroshock chair in your home, the programmer will carry a Taser kit. The perpetrators will say something like: "You will never be free." "Terminate your therapy." (Even if your therapist is a cult-planted therapist, your controllers might feel he or she has not closed you down sufficiently.) "You are a slave, nothing but a slave." "We will kill your child if you continue. You will not continue." Etc.

In regular life, your torturers may appear completely normal and non-cult-like. Some might hold high positions in society, such as doctors, lawyers, teachers, politicians, religious leaders. They might be your friends in daily life, or family members, or go to your church.

When you remember a recent punishment event, listen to their words carefully, because these will show their intent. Perpetrators will say something like stop your friendship with X, stop reading books about mind control, get off the online message board, stop talking about programs. If they cannot stop you from continuing in honest and authentic therapy, then they will program you to kill your therapist and/or yourself. They can order homicide through mind control. You, of course, do not have to do what they command.

All this abuse will occur during the early morning hours, when your unknowing neighbors sleep and do not call the police. The police on duty at these times very well may be cult-police plants. These groups excel in coordinating atrocities. Their break-ins often occur early on Saturday mornings, so you do not go to work drugged and with prominent bruises.

When you wake up from your drugged state later in the morning or afternoon, your mind probably will not recall what happened to you hours ago. This abuse can take place month after month or even week after week or day after day and still you will probably not recall it. The parts of your mind that are tortured are buried within your internal mind-control system, not easily accessible. If you do not find them and do not move far away, this kind of most vicious abuse can go on indefinitely. It can continue even if you move away. These groups are no respecters of age and frailty. It pays to dig and scratch and get to the parts who endured it and hear what they have to tell.

Even when your mind holds no conscious account of what recently occurred, your body can tell you. There is no way to endure this level of torture and not have a sore and injured body. If they think you might run away, they could break your foot or toes, or dislocate your knee or hip. Your torturers intend for you to be sore. If your mind is closed, ask your body. Follow the physical pain and ask inside about it. Much rides on your knowing what is happening to you and why. Try not to rationalize it away with some cause from normal life, like new orthotics or taking too long a hike. Knowing about your ongoing mind control is your best protection.

Their second kind of torture is for maintenance. For these, you will have to attend rituals. You will be instructed to travel to ritual sites. Rituals are for mind control. They have theatrical demonstrations, orgies, drugs, sometimes human sacrifices, and punishment for others. Their main purpose is to control your mind and keep you in place.

It is better to know what is happening to you.

It is better not to give your mind over.

It is better not to fold under their threats of harming someone you love.

They might have already harmed your pet.

Do not collapse under feelings of betrayal. One of the torturers they send may be one of your own mind-controlled children. That adult may torture your pet. The rest of that person will not know what he or she was forced to do.

Do not fold. Your mind belongs to you, not to your perpetrators. Your best protection is learning how your mind-control system works.

There might come a time when you realize that the body pains you suffer from are not body memories of years ago but fresh wounds. And the insomnia is not old anxiety but a fear of another assault. And the panic attacks are not amorphous and about your whole life but about specific fears concerning the here and now.

If you have reporters inside who have not stopped reporting to the abuser group, stay where you are until you are certain they will not report your plans. What is the sense of hiding if you are going to tattle on yourself? Before you can leave, you must spend your time finding all your inside reporters and enlighten them that they do not have to tell anyone where they are and that they can lie as well. They can report to you any danger they perceive instead.

Once it filters into your conscious mind that you are being accessed and beaten up brutally, electroshocked and drugged, there is only one way to cope. You have to leave. You cannot stay in your home or even your locality.

Even if you have family—especially if you have family—a nice job, friends, a church, clubs, you have to leave. You have to leave if you are twenty-five or seventy-five. Make careful plans, then take action.

Handlers*

Wendy Hoffman

If you are a mind-controlled victim, you are likely to have a handler until you escape or die. A handler makes sure you follow all commands, that your programs remain intact, that you make no moves toward breaking free. A handler can be a male or female adult. Handlers used to be called "manufacturers" because they manufacture your life and consider you a mannequin. They do not love you. They differ from programmers, who split off the personalities within you, and teach these parts the programs and commands. Programmers used to be called "mind masters." Often, parts are told they were "created" by the Master and, therefore, would not exist otherwise and belong to him. Sometimes the same person works as a programmer and a handler. Handlers also differ from spies, who follow you around to get information about you and snitch to the cult. They used to be called "snitches." And torturers work directly with programmers to administer the physical brutality. They can also be sent out on their own to enforce a program or threaten by giving a physical warning.

How do you get a handler?

---

* This chapter appeared in the online journal *Survivorship*, Winter 2016.

All cult-born people have one until they are trained. If they have specific ongoing jobs to do in their particular cult, then they will be assigned handlers to track their course. Because the danger of sudden enlightenment or programs breaking down lurks throughout a lifetime, handlers keep a vigilant eye on their subjects. Their jobs are made easy because victims are programmed to report promptly if something is not working within. So, even if handlers have lazy spells, are distracted, or miss a beat, their subjects will bring any indiscretion or striving for freedom to their handlers' attention. It is quite a *pas-de-deux*. A handler wants the complete slavery of his or her victims. The victims cooperate fully because they have been mind-controlled from infancy on to do so. They are not aware of this entrapment or of their programming to live as rats in a maze.

Like a pimp, the same handler can monitor many people's lives. But cult victims who have highly visible or important jobs in the normal, non-cult world will have a one-on-one handler. Handlers can be parents, siblings, spouses, lovers, relatives, friends, or therapists. I have seen heads of countries, royalty, and elected officials with their spouses on television, and it appeared to me that the spouses had been given the job of monitoring every action and thought of the officials they were in charge of and married to. Many of the people in charge of the world we live in are manipulated marionettes on tight strings. People in important visible positions will have solid handlers who will not deviate from their loyalty to the satanic cult. If they break free, these handlers will be demoted and punished.

You know you are in particular trouble when someone that parts of you recognize from your division of the cult enters your ordinary life. That can only mean one thing, and it does not mean your long lost love has somehow found you. It means your programmers are worried about your realizing who you are and have sent a more powerful and vicious handler to you, someone who knows you from the prior cult days even though most of your parts might not remember this person's true and secret identity.

People in less visible positions might have handlers who are also blind victims. Your breaking free might even help them see their own entrapment.

Breaking free of these prisons entails becoming aware that you are imprisoned. One reason you might not know you are entrapped is because of the tight reins handlers keep on their victims. No move toward awareness or freedom is tolerated. You can break free anyway.

Begin by identifying the current handler in your life.

If you have a compulsion to call somebody, that somebody would be your handler. You might call to report a move, some change in your life, a memory breaking out, or any information that goes against your programming.

If the handler is a friend or boss, you can gradually ease away, but what if the handler is a husband or wife and the parent of your child or children? You can divorce, but what do you do about the children? This is an instance of how complicated life becomes when attempting to extricate yourself from the webs of evil.

Some people may feel that they have to remain a prisoner because breaking away is too dangerous or difficult. If this is the case, it still might be better for you to know what your programs and triggers are than to go through life numb and deceived. If you know who your handler is, you can lie to that person. You do not have to report what you are thinking and feeling. You can be inching your way to freedom and perhaps preparing your child or children to make a break, while hiding this information from the now-known enemy.

When you are advanced in your recovery, a helpful therapeutic method is to make a list of the handlers you have had throughout your life. They may be few or many, depending on your age and your position in your criminal organization. Knowing what your life is and who the enemy is helps you regain the humanity that was stolen from you as soon as you were born. It is a way to give birth to yourself by pulling yourself away from people who plan to keep you down, who plan to make you less than a human being.

No matter how difficult the struggle is to break free, it is worth it. Moving in the right direction has its own rewards. Even if you cannot take your children with you, you are leaving them the legacy that the fight for freedom is worth it.

Your handler holds your programs like so many pebbles in his or her closed fist. You can start to open your brain, which will force your handler to drop the pebbles.

Called back

Wendy Hoffman

Reporter parts of survivors let perpetrators know, usually via a family member, if the survivors are remembering or telling secrets. Then the call-backs happen. Return to find out what people remember. Return to get revenge. Return because granddad is dying. Etcetera. When a survivor returns to her cult family, she will most likely be tortured with electroshock, raped, and reprogrammed to know nothing about her secret life. Her amnesic barriers will be repaired and resurrected.

Survivors remember going home merrily to celebrate birthdays, parents' anniversaries, siblings' graduations, marriages, funerals, major holidays—the usual. They returned to visit someone hospitalized. Some family ties remained, so they had to participate. Then comes the bitter realization that they remember the before and after but not the event they were called home for, perhaps a ritual, with torture, drugs, and commands. Perhaps one of the survivor's programs had started to slip. Perhaps the person did not act according to schedule. Perhaps they did not respond promptly enough to telephone calls and emails. All that was repaired through torturous mind control during these imposed "visits" and "reunions".

When I started my memory process, I compulsively went back to my childhood neighborhood, planning to talk to people who lived there to see whether they had seen or heard anything which could have led them to suspect I had been an abused child. I was unaware that I followed a "return home" program. In my childhood neighborhood, I underwent torture and my mind was re-erased by those still living there. What I would have given to have been warned. Even if I did not listen, I would have known someone on the outside world cared. I believe I would have listened. It would have saved decades of my life.

If you are a survivor, do not be taken in by either your family's apparently warm invitations or your inner urgings to go home. If your family is cult, just do not go.

What do you do if you are a therapist who follows the rules and your client wants to cancel sessions for a while and go home to the family she grew up in? This client does not know yet about programming to return home when you start having memories. And her front person feels excited about seeing the family again.

As a therapist, you do not want to suggest. If the trip home is successful by cult standards, she will remember nothing and stop treatment. There may or may not be a second chance for her to have therapy to help dismantle the mind control. You can take the conservative approach and ask how the client feels about seeing her family again, whether she has any misgivings, whether anyone inside has reported that she is in therapy and working on remembering and associating.

You can target questions so that they bypass the front person who knows nothing and goes straight to the inside parts. "How do you feel about returning home?" Maybe one of the inside parts will pop through the amnesiac barriers to answer truthfully and say "Do not." But maybe not. Then it may be the moment to switch aim and address the front person directly. Who cares about suggesting? This human being might never get another chance at freedom.

Speaking as a survivor, I think this is the moment to tell the front person about "return home" programming. You can say it gently. It does not have to be hit-over-the-head direct, though sometimes that is the only way front people hear necessary information. But information should be conveyed even if it will not be listened to. At least you tried. Maybe the victim will hear it a decade later.

Therapeutic rules were not designed for war, or for life and death situations. There's a time to be cautious and a time to be bold. This might be the only chance. There are more important issues than correct therapeutic procedure. Safety comes first.

Why and how survivors are gathered

Alison Miller

In the years since I have been treating survivors of mind control and ritual abuse, there has been a great flowering of resources for these survivors. Websites with discussion boards on which survivors can talk about their experiences, coping strategies, and attempts at healing; first-person accounts of being victimized; books promising cures; Facebook discussion groups; conferences for survivors; support networks; safe houses.

What do all these things mean? Are we to rejoice that so many resources exist? Or are we to be wary? I would say the latter. We have to worry about more than disinformation. Any venue that brings together survivors of these abuses brings them into contact with persons who are able to access their programming through pre-arranged signals or cues, and set off various kinds of programs. One of my earliest experiences with this occurred when a well-known survivor who has written books visited Vancouver, along with her rescuer, who may have been her handler. At this event, which hundreds of people attended, we were all asked to fill out the Dissociative Experiences Scale, and use a pseudonym as our identity. At the end of their talk, they read out a supposed list of the pseudonyms of people who should be concerned about their dissociation. My colleague and I realized that these were just strings of letters and numbers, probably intended to trigger programming, plus those people were asked to remain behind to receive further "help."

I had another such experience in the mid-1990s when a well-known ritual abuse expert came to our area, and all the therapists attended his talk. Mine was one of the British Columbia locations where he spoke. Stella Katz (the former cult programmer who contributed to my books) attended, and told me he was wearing a ring which indicated very high cult rank, a ring which she had seen only once before. A client of mine became a quivering little childish ball of fear, saying only that she had seen him before and he was bad and had hurt her. And I heard him in the hotel elevator humming the tune of a nursery rhyme that I knew to be a trigger to cause an internal "earthquake" in survivors' personality systems, thrusting those systems into chaos.

This man announced that we could tell whether our phones were being tapped by calling a certain number in California; if we got a busy signal, it meant our phones were tapped. Afterwards, one enterprising therapist from another town, where he had said the same thing, contacted the California telephone company and they traced that phone number to a locked office from where it gave a perpetual busy signal. Our then network of therapists cancelled the rest of his tour.

Conferences can be wonderful places where survivors can learn from one another and from helpful speakers. But they can also be places where survivors are accessed by perpetrator group members and re-abused, including survivors who were physically safe prior to the conference. Perpetrator attendees or speakers can use hand signals or trigger words or visual images like tarot cards or playing cards to bring out compliant parts and trigger programs. They can knock on hotel room doors at night with patterned knocks designed to get a child part or an unsafe roommate to open the door, and then enter and abuse the survivor.

Perhaps online discussion groups might be safer. But not necessarily. If members are permitted to share personal information with other members, that information can be reported to perpetrator groups. Members can invite others to stay with them for conferences, and bad things can happen during such visits. Even online, words can be used to trigger programming. I do not have much experience with many of these websites or discussion groups, but I have enough to have seen this in action. "Matriarchs" gather members under their wing, providing what the members believe to be support, but actually keeping those survivors in line through the use of words and phrases with double meanings. An article on one website for survivors pooh-poohs the idea that hand signals and other triggers are real and can have actual effects on survivors, suggesting that those who talk about this are spreading paranoia and can lead survivors to go crazy. Some articles on such websites are very helpful; others include coded messages reinforcing programming and disinformation.

I know that survivors are lonely for others who understand their suffering and their attempts to find freedom. Recovery is a lonely journey. But loneliness is better than continued abuse. Survivors, be careful.

Danger, DANGER

Wendy Hoffman

Like hospitals and therapists, some safe houses for survivors are safe and some are not. It is up to survivors to use as much good judgment and discernment as possible before taking refuge in a safe house.

When I was banished from Canada, I was about to go out on my own. A woman telephoned Alison, saying she and a colleague were driving through Victoria, and requested an interview with her. The couple said they had a ritually abused friend, and wanted help in how to support her and other survivors of such abuses. They had started an organization to help people in this field. Alison thought they seemed sincere, so she asked if I could have safe temporary housing with them while I looked for a place to live. I was not overjoyed, but Alison was excited. She did not want to see me drive out into the blue yonder alone. I felt she was over-confident, though I did not tell her this. Eventually, I decided to go to them, though I had never met them and Alison had only met them this once. Despite Alison's enthusiasm and my trust in her, I think I might have resisted this ominous offer had other programmers not broken into my house and given me instructions to contact this disguised woman and take up residence there while I looked for permanent housing, or they would murder

Alison. I wondered why I changed my mind so abruptly. It was not that I reconsidered. It was programming. Watch for swift changes of mind in yourself.

The only thing that bothered me from the beginning was that this was all so coincidental. Once, when I lived in New York City, I was excited about meeting someone new and told my then Israeli handler, whom I did not know, of course, was a handler. He asked how I had met this person. I told him just by lucky chance. He shook his head. That is how I learned that in this world of bad mind control, serendipity and good coincidences do not occur, only awful set-ups.

When I arrived at the small, compact home in a western city, I met the woman, who had read, underlined, and studied my first memoir. She was an emaciated, perfumed woman with long red dyed hair and lots of make-up, married to a tall and rather obedient accountant. She talked constantly, was warm and outgoing. I would not have been able to tell she is an enforcer and torturer.

The husband and her colleague, the other male who made the initial visit to Alison, were present. We talked for a while. Then—I'll call her Liz—Liz insisted she and I go out for dinner, though I was exhausted. Later, I went to sleep. In the earliest hours of morning, they woke me, dragged me onto the floor and began the routine torture and enforcing that would go on for the seven weeks I was in residence there. Most of their commands were never to be in therapy again, not ever to write again, not to remember the new torture-based mind control. And I did not for a long time. Once a week, they drugged me and took me to an office building downtown where I had programming in electroshock chairs in the basement of psychiatrists' offices. Their overseer came by at least once a week. He had access to my computerized black books, where most of my programming information is stored. People are walking around with it now in their cell phones.

This effusive, anorexic woman did not seem cult-like, and neither did her tight male partner in their organization, or her friendly but blank husband, or their one personable adult son. Their other son, however, did show signs.

I could not tell, Alison could not, a sharp administrator for one of the conferences on dissociation (whose antennae are always outstretched) could not tell. Much later, I remembered having seen this couple attend mind control survivors' conferences and reprogram people there. I believe they go on assignment to targeted survivors who are high up in the cult hierarchy, or healing well and have something to give back to survivors and the world. We were all duped, even though this mind control team is not particularly bright. The ramifications are just awful.

A long time ago, in the 1950s, a Nazi group stole and sequestered three of my thirteen original split infants. These current Nazi programmers had the information about where these parts of me were hidden internally. They knew how to call them out. If you have even one infant who has not been incorporated into the main healed mind, then perpetrators can build on that part. That is what happened to me.

Besides my caution of danger, danger, this is all I can suggest: Survivors have been trained in psychic awareness, some more, some less. Engage your far-sighted psychic vision. With your inner eyes, observe the exterior of the person under scrutiny. Now use your internal energy to cut through the surface. Do you bump into an ice block, a core of frozenness that is frightening and off-putting? Do you see a narcissism (a sense of self-importance) that goes way beyond ordinary-life narcissism? Do you see a confusion of mind? These perpetrators often think they are helping their victims have better lives. If you see such characteristics, stay away. Perhaps you just see that the outside and inside do not match. If you go deeper, you may find a severely wounded child. Do not let that distract you. You are not there to rescue this person, you are there to assess. Where there is ice, self-involvement, and confusion, there may be a perpetrator, no matter what the surface projects and no matter how hurt the person may be. Do not take any chances. A suspicion is sufficient for stopping the relationship.

In addition, do not trust coincidences. Chances are, they were planted and you were targeted.

Do not give over your mind to someone else, no matter how much that person desires to help you and is also an expert. It would be lovely not to have to make all these important decisions alone, but it is only you who knows what is best for you, mind control or not. Often, it is safest to be alone.

Danger lurks out there, especially as you restore your self.

Discarding the interventionist God

Alison Miller

The length of time Wendy was allowed to stay in Canada was coming to an end, and I was quite worried about her return to the USA. To my knowledge, she had not experienced any abuse during the year she had been in Canada, and she and I often speculated about why that might be. Of course, we did not know that some of her previous perpetrators had made several visits to her, pulling out a small group of parts she had not yet discovered. And they knew when she was going to have to leave.

When the American woman, "Liz," from the fairly new support organization, contacted me, I was happy to meet her, and in the back of my mind was the possibility that these "supporters" could help Wendy through her next move. When I met Liz and her rather taciturn business partner, they seemed rather naïve but genuinely concerned. They said they were Christians who wanted to help survivors, including a woman they named as their friend. The timing, and the fact that they came all the way from the city they lived in to my place in Victoria, should have made me suspicious, but they did not. I took a leap of faith and asked them about the possibility of their helping Wendy (whose name I did not yet give them, of course) in exchange for my helping them support their survivor friend and speaking at a conference they were organizing.

I had grown up with honest, thoughtful, kind and gentle parents, and in benign and encouraging schools, so despite working with survivors of horrendous abuses, my natural tendency was to expect people to be good and to be what they said they were. Plus, somewhere deep in my own soul was a longing for the interventionist God I had believed in for at least twenty years beginning at the age of fifteen.

Could that God have sent people just at the right time? Oh, what a wonderful happy ending that would be. Somehow, it did not occur to me that those people might indeed have been sent, but not by Him. Although I do not remember our conversations on this topic, Wendy tells me that I encouraged her to trust the people who had said they were willing to take her in, assuming she was just responding from an automatic tendency to distrust even well-meaning people. I did not know she was going against an instinct that might have kept her safe.

Do not trust your therapist too fully; he or she is only human. The reality that your therapist is a decent human being and can be relied upon to care about you does not mean that he or she knows everything, especially about the dangers in this world. I am deeply saddened by Wendy's further abuse at the hands of people who appeared kind. Therapists, like their clients, are affected by their own past experiences. Those like me who are not child abuse survivors can all too easily see the world with rose-colored glasses. Those who are survivors, especially of mind control and ritual abuse, can all too easily grasp at straws to find a faith that will sustain them as they gradually become aware of what horrendous things they have endured.

How do we make sense of it all? Here are some things most people believe:

1. Good and evil exist, and we make choices about them.
2. There is a God who is good and loving.
3. God is also all-powerful.
4. Horrible things happen.

Mind control and ritual abuse are atrocities, and, to those of us who know about them, there is no doubt that they happen, and on a much larger scale than I ever imagined. How can such things happen, if a loving God has power over everything? Trying to make sense of these things, people come up with beliefs, such as:

- *Victims deserve what happens to them, because they are evil.* The abuser groups pound this idea into their victims' heads from day one. I cannot accept that an infant whose hand is used to stab a drugged victim is evil, or that someone who chooses the lesser of two evils is, therefore, evil, when no good choice exists.
- *Victims are being repaid by the law of karma for evil that they did in past lives.* It is easy for a ritual abuse survivor to believe this about him or herself, and I have known survivors who believed it, in order to make God and the universe just. But what about the African babies who are born with HIV, or the millions of people who died in the Holocaust and other genocides? More people have endured these horrors in the past century than the number of human beings who inhabited the earth before them, so the numbers do not work, if suffering in this life is a penalty for misbehavior in a past life.
- *God, in his love, sends ritual abuse as a special gift to purify the soul of victims.* I actually heard this one spoken by a "Christian" survivor therapist at a conference, and I walked out. What kind of God would do this? Perhaps this speaker did not realize how horrendous these abuses are. Her God was not a loving one.

Ritualistic abusers tell a little child to pray and see whether God comes to help. Of course, God does not show up. Then they suggest she call on Satan, and of course, the man in the red suit appears. Now she knows that either God is not loving, or God regards her as not worth saving, or God is helpless, or God just does not care, or God does not exist. And history shows us that God just does not stick his finger in and prevent atrocities from happening, even though the victors in all wars say God helped them. (Bob Dylan wrote a great song about that—*With God on our Side.*)

The only way I can make sense of atrocities and still believe in a loving God is by accepting that God does not intervene in human affairs in any direct manner. I have to discard the interventionist God, and I have to resist being lured into hoping that God is intervening, and remember that "When something seems too good to be true, it probably is." Believing in an interventionist God is dangerous. It can lead to passivity rather than active resistance against evil, and waiting around for help rather than helping ourselves. It can also lead us to trust people who are not trustworthy.

My alternatives are: Believe there is no God, or believe in a God who does not intervene, not because s/he is unwilling, but because the universe just doesn't work that way. Atheists and agnostics can still make moral choices, and choose kindness over evil, like the doctor in Albert Camus's famous novel *The Plague*.

I choose to hope that there is a God who loves, and who suffers with those who suffer, as we therapists suffer with our clients, even though He does not directly intervene. It is not a certainty, only a hope, based on survivors' near-death experiences and my own inner sense of connecting to a compassion within the core of me which might be beyond myself.

When they persist in trying to murder you . . .

Wendy Hoffman

I do not think that I am the only one whom perpetrators hound, attempt to trigger, and pursue.

Alison tells me that they let several of her clients go even before she met them, so that she could work with them freely as long as they did not report back to their group. She says that they made a deal with another, something like "freedom for silence." But that has not happened to me. I would not agree to silence at any rate. If I had the opportunity to make a deal, I would refuse it.

They pursue people like me who want to give back to other survivors and help repair the world.

Their preferred method is to make homicide look like suicide. They come into your home while the world sleeps and call out vulnerable inside parts. An intruder pries open the victim's mouth and another spills a bottle of lethal pills down his or her throat. That is probably the most common method. Alison tells me that two of her first group of survivor clients reported this kind of attempt to her, and, in *Healing the Unimaginable* (Chapter One), she describes the probable murder of a third, who supposedly climbed out her eighth floor window though she was too fat and weak to do so. I, too, had an ex-client who jumped out of a high window after men dressed as firemen entered her apartment. People in that community think it was a homicide.

Or they can break into your home, slit your wrists and make it look like suicide. If you have made prior suicide attempts, this is a bonus for the perpetrators, because investigators are likely to assume your death is suicide rather than murder. Murderers will call out a suicidal part before the homicide occurs, so that the victim will not struggle or make a noise.

Alison also tells me that they used to sneak up on her clients, drug them by putting a rag over their faces from behind, and drag them into a van. She cautions me to stay clear of cars so that I am not dragged into one. In the vans, they usually only torture but may also murder. I have had men sneak up on me and shove a gun into my back, then threaten me using code words.

Some of their methods of homicide are more indirect. They can tamper with your car, or enlist one of their suicide soldiers to drive into your car. Or they can push you off a bridge, order you to jump off a bridge, shoot you as you take a pleasant, normal kind of walk in a park (one of their sniper soldiers can do that).

You might have lunch with a good "friend" whom you do not suspect yet. That friend may easily slip poison into your food when you go to the bathroom or even look away for a moment. I was taught how to do this at political parties. They can also substitute your medications for poisoned meds that look the same. They even contaminate supplements. They place two cyanide tablets on the top of your bottle of supplements or vitamins. Cyanide and other poisons can be fashioned to look the same as your usual pills.

I am telling you these methods so that you can be aware. It is frightening but so much safer to know. If you remain oblivious, you are more of a sitting duck. Your best defense is to know every part of your brain that has been separated and named through mind control.

Another injustice is that the perpetrators have your "black book" with almost complete information on the parts, their names, how to call them out, their purpose, ages, and triggers. And you only have your recovery process and possibly a safe therapist who will not know so much about your mind control as the readers of your "black book." The more parts you have knowledge of, the safer you will be. You can take them out of where programmers told them to live and move them to a new and healthy living environment—all done internally though you might have to change your external location as well.

If you always hated the group and did not want to join them, they might be after you. Since it is so very difficult to know who is safe and whom to trust, it is probably better not to confide in anyone until you are sure of the person, and you may never be sure. If you are absolutely sure that someone is safe, and you can tolerate living with someone, that protection might make you safer. But mind-controlled people can never really be absolutely sure. There could still be some part in your brain that has not told what happened. So it is wise always to be suspicious. How did you meet this "safe" person? Is this person connected to anyone in your cult? Some people have safe and courageous friends. Most do not. I do have three non-survivor friends who are safe and courageous. However, I was accessed on one of their properties. They did not know, of course.

Make a list of all your known perpetrators. You can have a section for suspected perpetrators whom you do not have memories about (yet?). People in survivors' worlds are usually cult. Better to be wary than murdered or even tortured and re-programmed. This process is long enough without further difficulties. All this reprogramming takes time to unravel, time taken away from when you might have a real life. Healing is not only finding your parts one group after the other, but also disengaging from your monitors and programmers, one contact person after the other.

Expect a lot of triggering communication. At least one of your "friends" will monitor your location and emotional mood. That person will scan you for traces of straining at the leash and wanting to be free. If you disappear even for a weekend, expect emails asking where you are. Also expect requests for favors. Another "friend" may want you to drive her or him somewhere. That will be a set-up to get you to a specific location, where others may be waiting.

A long distance "friend" may request to visit you. Say no. The emails will have trigger words that pull out vulnerable parts inside you. Actually, expect constant harassment. Expect guns, and look for the parts inside you that obey when they see a gun pointed at them or pressed into them even in a public place where there is no likelihood that the person will actually shoot it. Expect the worst and stay safe. Do not become over-confident if you have months or years of peace and non-harassment. Eventually, they might check up on you. Some survivors feel guilty about endangering other people who are helping them. There is no doubt that this is a horrendously dangerous field.

However, you are giving non-cult people the opportunity to be more decent as human beings. There is more to life than making yourself as comfortable as possible and making your children's lives as cushy as possible.

Keep fighting the criminals who harass you, keep fighting even if the criminals are your family.

The proximity of death raises questions of whether life is worth it. People with easy lives will be happy to preach to you. It is your decision alone. One of the benefits of not dying is that you are then still fighting them. Our purpose in being alive is not only to eat chocolate cake but also to help others and to make the world more free of evil.

Spy school: clues we missed

Alison Miller

I have said before that this is psychologically sophisticated organized crime. It is sophisticated in the way its trainers or programmers subdivide a child's brain through torture and threats, so that they can make that child do what they want, including things that are completely contradictory to that child's nature. It is particularly sophisticated in its security. Victims, for the most part, do not know they are victims, and do not know what has happened to them. Their family and closest friends can be perpetrators, and they will not know it. A victim can be tortured one night and go to therapy the next day and not remember what happened during the night!

External security is also sophisticated. Perpetrator group members deliberately infiltrate the systems that are designed to protect the vulnerable. That means they are among the police, among hospital staff (particularly mental hospitals), among therapists (psychologists, social workers, counselors), among physicians (particularly psychiatrists), among staff of non-profit agencies. The fox is guarding the henhouse.

Most of us who work in these settings are unaware that some of our colleagues might be members of such a group. Some of those colleagues who are group members might be conscious of it; others might be used unwittingly, as Wendy was when working as a therapist, a story she tells in *The Enslaved Queen* (2014). This is one of the things I do not want to know, but there it is. Wendy did not want to know it either—but she was willing to know it, and I was willing to hear it.

How do you know whether a person is a member of a perpetrator group? He or she will not come up to you and announce it, unless you are a dissociative survivor and the group member can give a cue to switch you to a compliant part, whose experiences you will not remember later. As we wrote in some previous essays, we had the awful experience of Wendy being in the hands of perpetrators, and being unaware of it.

Over the years of dealing with survivors and with colleagues, I saw many little clues that someone might possibly be a perpetrator group member or, at least, a victim, but I did not put them together until later. Here are some of the clues I remember as I look back. No one of these clues means much on its own, like the symptoms on a checklist, but put together they might alert us to be a bit suspicious.

Knowing too much about mind control, or ritual abuse, or dissociation, or about abuser networks

If a person demonstrates knowledge about mind control, ritual abuse, dissociation, or abuser networks that he or she would not normally be expected to have, you need to be alert and cautious. How would that person have obtained that information? If it is possible without arousing that person's suspicion, ask how he or she knows that. Perhaps it is innocent, but perhaps the knowledge comes from inside experience.

Example: A local junior trainee therapist spoke up in a Mental Health Center staff meeting when we were discussing a teenage boy I was treating. She suggested he might have a dissociative disorder. At that time, nobody knew about dissociative disorders—so why did she? I later discovered she was a cult member (when a relative of hers approached me for therapy, and disclosed to me the therapist's involvement).

Example: I was looking for local therapists whom I could train in working with mind control survivors. Someone I knew suggested another therapist in her own support group who had read my *Healing the Unimaginable* and recommended it to her to help with a client she was treating. I accepted supervision of the therapist, who seemed keen, though she said she had never had a survivor client before. I sent her a high-functioning ritual abuse survivor client. The client emailed me a few months later saying she had quit seeing the therapist, who was repeatedly missing sessions or cancelling at the last minute. It might be that the therapist was herself an unknowing survivor. Why would she have read my book if she had never seen such a client?

Example: A supposedly healed survivor who had spoken at a conference told me that the conference organizer had invited her (and me, the previous year) to speak as "the draw," in order to get survivors to attend and be accessed and reprogrammed. I had never heard of this technique with regard to conferences. I later heard evidence that the "healed" survivor was herself a plant, an active perpetrator. As the old saying goes, "it takes one to know one."

Seeming to know too little about areas in which they claim expertise

Sometimes people "pad" their resumés to appear to know things they do not really know. In other cases, like the examples below, people know far more than they want to let on that they know. Cult insiders may want to appear ignorant of such matters.

Example: A detective who said he was developing a model for how to investigate ritual abuse cases presented a muddled plan which involved only very basic police work, suitable for finding a little backwoods cult, not a sophisticated network. I wondered why he seemed to know so little. Wendy later discovered the hard way that he was a perpetrator.

Example: His business partner, who worked with sexual abuse survivors, initially refused to believe me when I told her that someone she had recommended to help a survivor had actually abused the survivor. When I told her that the survivor had reported that the woman had sexually assaulted her, the person who worked with sexual assault cases appeared shocked because I mentioned sex. Why would this be shocking to someone in such a profession, or to anyone who knew anything at all about mind control and ritual abuse?

Too much forgetfulness

Many factors, including illness and fatigue, can contribute to forgetting. But when people frequently forget conversations and agreements they should have remembered, it can be a sign of dissociation. This does not mean they are part of a perpetrator group, but it raises the possibility that they have been victimized and might be used by such a group. Or that they are trying to deceive you. Or that they are perpetrators trying to deceive you.

Lack of compassion, operating from just intellect

Higher-up perpetrator-identified parts in victims have been trained to have no emotions, the emotions being held by hidden child parts. They simply speak and act as they have been told to do. If a person you know goes into such a state, it might indicate that such a part is operating. "Conscious" perpetrators might be this way, with occasional episodes of raging frenzy when the emotions break through. Wendy tells me that she remembers at least four different master programmers having meltdowns and psychotic breaks during programming sessions, starting with her grandfather, Max and Mengele.

Example: The local therapist trainee who turned out to be a cult member co-facilitated a therapy group for teenagers with me. The group was always very quiet, as the trainee therapist, who was the primary leader, seemed to follow a rigid plan rather than being flexible in responding to the members' needs. She felt to me as if she had a block of ice at her core, cold and unreachable. When she left the center and turned the group over to me, the members immediately bonded and began to open up with one another—but not until she was gone.

All four of the cult-involved therapists that Wendy went to before she found me fitted into this category. One treated everyone like a specimen, one was very judgmental and looked down on people, one was very self-righteous, and one was extremely self-centered. Wendy's front person saw glimpses of pleasure when they lied to her, frustrated her, or made her feel stupid. The one who was a cult programmer took particular delight in torturing and demeaning her.

Becoming rigidly attached to a certain approach; speaking in a manner as if reciting without tolerating interruption

People with brain damage, and people who are highly emotionally triggered, may do this. Some people in an emotional state can only think in a linear manner, and need to control the conversation in this way. However, some people doing this might be speaking from programming, using words they have memorized and have to speak in the order they heard them. Sometimes, such people are just victims rather than perpetrators. I have learned to use this clue to recognize when a survivor I am speaking with is speaking from programming rather than thinking independently. Persons who are part of perpetrator groups believe the lies the groups told them, and are likely to speak memorized lies.

Example: Two cult-involved therapists that Wendy went to were hyper-religious, putting forth their supposedly Christian religious beliefs in a very self-centered manner rather than tuning in to the client.

Twisting the truth about other people, accusing people you know are innocent of being perpetrators or plants

The community of those who attempt to help survivors is constantly suffering from splits as some accuse others of having nefarious motives. When I hear such things, I have learned to look at the accuser first rather than the accused.

Example: The supposedly healed survivor whom I mentioned under the first subheading above accused a number of other speakers at the conference where she had given a talk of being part of the perpetrator group. Some of those speakers are respected clinicians whom I know well enough to be quite sure they are not perpetrators, even though the fact that someone is a respected clinician does not guarantee he or she is not a perpetrator.

Example: A clinician I knew well went on sabbatical, and handed a survivor client over to another clinician at her workplace. Within a short time the client, backed by her new therapist, was making outrageous allegations against her former therapist, a person I know personally to be someone of great integrity. The collaboration with the new therapist, who would have no way of substantiating the allegations against her colleague, makes me more suspicious of the new therapist than of the client, who would be simply believing deceptions of the perpetrator group.

Example: Wendy had personal experience of several politicians being involved in mind control. One of Wendy's cult-involved therapists told Wendy's front person, disdainfully, that one politician was "the satanic pick," while saying that another, whom other parts of Wendy had seen at the Feast of the Beast, was a good man. In retrospect, it showed Wendy that the one accused by the therapist must be a less evil man.

Making accusations against one another to confuse you

Perpetrators who are in cahoots often pretend to dislike one another. They may accuse one another of being cult plants, thereby demonstrating their own apparent innocence. Do not be deceived by this. Remember that the fact that if someone accuses someone else of being a perpetrator, it does not mean that the accuser is not a perpetrator, even if the person accused is one.

Example: Wendy's cult-assigned boyfriend pretended he did not like the cult-assigned therapist with whom he worked as a team. Wendy's programmer therapist frequently said bad things to Wendy about her assistant programmers and her cult-assigned boyfriend.

Example: The "healed survivor" who spoke at the conference made accusations against everyone associated with that conference, not all of whom were innocent. The innocent and the guilty were put in the same package in her accusations.

Entitled, demanding, or demeaning behavior

In general, it is wise to watch out for people who want to use you for their own ends. This is even more true of "conscious" members of organized perpetrator groups. Such people tend to be narcissistic, to look down on survivors, and to need power. Wendy reports that all four of her cult-involved therapists were like this. If someone shows these characteristics, be suspicious. Be especially suspicious if they give orders that a survivor instantly obeys. Wendy, on the basis of her own experience, says: "When a survivor gets up and starts mindlessly following directions she doesn't want to, it is probably mind control. It would be fine to scream at the survivor, snap fingers in her face, shake her. Anything to bring her back to consciousness."

Example: When Wendy left Canada and stayed for seven weeks with the "helpful" woman I sent her to, she told me that she was doing all the woman's shopping, cooking, and housework and paying for all the food. I thought this was odd, but did not put two and two together. I assumed that Wendy must have offered to help out, and the woman had accepted her offer instead of asking her to pay rent. I knew that Wendy's mother had always had a cleaning lady, and, consequently, Wendy had always had one, too. Wendy herself did not catch on to what was happening, because of dissociation. The woman turned out to be a perpetrator, and Wendy's housework behavior, inconsistent with her nature and habits, was programmed obedience. I should have noticed.

Example: Wendy flew to another city to hear me present a day-long workshop for therapists. She and I returned on the same flight. I was to have a long layover in the airport where she was disembarking, and she told me that she would stay with me for a few hours before driving to her destination. The same woman in the previous example had Wendy's car, and Wendy was to call to be picked up. When we had been in the airport a very short time, the woman phoned Wendy and told her to come and be picked up immediately. Wendy obeyed instantly, though she grumbled to me. I was quite surprised. I assumed that she did not want to inconvenience the woman, who had apparently looked at the flight schedule, seen when the plane would arrive, and gone to the airport rather than waiting for Wendy's call. I did not recognize what Wendy's instant obedience indicated: that the woman was a handler and Wendy was headed not to a pleasant drive home but to a torture session. I did not stop her.

Over-friendliness, appearing to have too much in common with you, or flattering you

Even when you are not dealing with people involved in organized perpetrator groups, over-friendliness should raise questions. One woman in my housing complex has used little bags of chocolates on festive occasions, leaving them at people's doors with a nice little note. Why? She is a realtor and she wants our business. Although the rest of my new neighbors are reasonably friendly, they do not invite me into the center of their friendship groups. They continue with their existing friends, and I with mine. If someone does not, they are after something. If you are a mind control victim, or a therapist for victims, and someone tries to be your best buddy, ask yourself what they might want.

Since I am not dissociative, I cannot be accessed through hand signals or other triggers. I cannot be tortured and mind-controlled to forget it. However, I can be deceived. When someone within my network of therapists and survivors tries to get close to me, flatters me, or praises me too much, and echoes what I say rather than stating their own views, I wonder why they are trying to manipulate me. Although I do not mind well-deserved appreciation, flattery is something different; it means the person has an ulterior motive. The flattery may speak about something realistic, but its intent is to manipulate.

Example: A woman contacted me via LinkedIn. Although she had a different identity on LinkedIn, she named herself as a well-known internet blogger who helped break open knowledge about ritual abuse and mind control. The original blogger, whose work has frequently helped my understanding, disappeared several years ago and there is speculation regarding whether she is dead or in hiding. The woman claiming to be her was inviting me to view her new website, which purported to be a continuation of the original person's blog. I asked her a number of questions about her background and how she'd managed to keep safe all those years, and how she had originally been used by the major perpetrator group. Her creative answers about her background did not fit with what the original person had written several years ago. She appears to be an impersonator, which means the original blogger is probably dead, or no one would claim to be her, and the new website is probably one to be avoided, especially by survivors.

Example: A supposedly healed survivor dropped my name and misquoted me in a blog post on her website, saying "I was just chatting with Alison Miller," as if we were the best of buddies. The fact was that I had spoken with her by telephone for perhaps ten minutes, and we had never met in person. The rest of the blog post promoted an approach to healing with which I thoroughly disagree. I felt used, and put in a response to the post indicating that I had been misquoted. My response was erased, and I am now on that website on the list of services to be avoided.

Example: When Wendy moved to a new location, several women immediately became friends with her, inviting her into their circle and engaging in activities with her. From a distance, I marvelled at the way she was able to make friends so quickly, unlike me in my new location. It turns out that my neighbors are normal. Wendy's friendship group members turned out to be on assignment from you-know-whom.

Perpetrator groups assign friends, boyfriends, and girlfriends to survivors in order to control them. Wendy remembers a programmer telling her to get rid of a boyfriend, saying "You are not allowed to have a boyfriend unless we send him to you." When a survivor is alone and becoming rebellious, what could be better than a potential partner, sent with the right moves to become intimate with the lonely and isolated survivor and become his or her new handler?

Example: Wendy produced and performed the play *INCEST: Remember & Tell*, and suddenly an old boyfriend, the one assigned by the cult to be the "king" to her queen, appeared in her life. He wormed his way into her play, changing things to its detriment, ousting her from her television spots and usurping her audiences. He came into her life to silence her and to pull her followers away from her.

Unexpected rudeness

When someone who has become friendly with you suddenly attacks you or cuts you off, you are taken aback and understandably confused. It can indicate that the person's friendliness was actually acting, something perpetrators are pretty good at, and they have become tired of doing it. Survivors are likely to take this rejection personally rather than scrutinizing the other person's motives.

Example: Not too long after Wendy moved away from a recent group of torturers, the woman who had hosted her suddenly blocked her emails, presumably because she was tired of trying to maintain the superficial side of the relationship. She denied having done it.

Example: A woman in a poetry workshop whom Wendy thought was a new friend read Wendy's memoir and then told Wendy she should never have written such a thing and that she was full of darkness. This statement reinforced all Wendy's programming about being evil and being unacceptable to normal people. Wendy discovered some time later that this was actually not a normal person, but the head of a local coven.

Coincidental timing

When something happens just at the right time, it might not be divine providence, and it might not be a happy coincidence. It might be the result of planning on the part of perpetrators. When people come out of nowhere and seem to have a great deal in common with you, or to have just the expertise you need, be cautious.

Example: I wanted somewhere safe for Wendy to stay when she left here, and "support people" showed up just at the right time. I thought it was divine providence. It was not. They had formed this support organization in order to access survivors for no good purpose.

Example: A local therapist approached me to become one of the associates in my practice. Unlike my known associates, she expressed an interest in working with survivors of mind control and ritual abuse. Of course, I received many more such referrals than I could take, so I would be happy to find someone who was willing to take on the challenge of this work. I presented this woman's credentials to my existing associates. Fortunately, one of them knew a great deal about her history, information which was not on her resumé, enough to make me suspect that she might be at least a survivor of such abuses and possibly an active member of a perpetrator group. I did not accept her.

Some of these examples are from my own life, some from Wendy's. Each of these "little things" I wondered at, but I did not wonder hard enough. I did not want to be paranoid. I was brought up to think the best of other people. People who appear to be helpers, who are dedicated to caring for those who have been hurt—how could I be suspicious of them? But I should have been.

I recently said to Wendy, "I never went to spy school." And she replied, "This *is* spy school." Reader, welcome to spy school.

SECTION VI

THE SURVIVOR'S DAILY LIFE

Ask inside

Alison Miller

Survivors of criminal abuse including mind control can be triggered into unpleasant emotional states and false beliefs even when their programming is no longer operating. If you have not processed all your traumatic memories, you are vulnerable without realizing it to being influenced by emotions and beliefs from your inside parts, emotions and beliefs which belong to the parts' past experiences rather than to the present.

A survivor was functioning well in a challenging workplace for which she had been required to provide a Criminal Record Check from the police. This would have been a simple statement that she had no criminal record—that is, according to the police she had never committed a crime. She had managed it satisfactorily the first time, going to the police station and getting a sealed envelope from the front desk and giving it to her supervisor. But several years later, the supervisor approached her and told her that the workplace had lost her Criminal Record Check, and they would like her to provide another. She became really upset, and the supervisor tried to joke with her about how she must be hiding some criminal activity, which only made things worse. She became convinced that her supervisor was out to get her. She would not listen to me when I said that there was no risk here. She did, however, permit me to ask the insiders in her personality system whether there was any memory regarding police. And, of course, she had the usual anti-police programming: As a child she had been taken by cult people dressed as police to an apparent police station where she was locked in a cell, told she was a criminal, and abused, and told that if she ever talked to the police this is what would happen to her again. I explained to her internal leaders that this was a cult trick, and that the Criminal Record Check was simply a brief statement that she (as an adult) had never been arrested for any crime. It would simply be picking up an envelope, just as it had been previously.

A survivor client of mine had been clean and sober for many years, but had previously had a drinking problem. She reported to me, with great embarrassment and shame, that she was coming home from work and drinking because the stress of her workplace was too great. I attempted without success to deal with this by finding her healthy relaxing activities she could engage in when she got home. It did not help. So I asked her inner children. It turned out that the source of the problem had nothing to do with the workplace. The adult had been searching online for children's cartoons and films which her child parts could watch on her computer. Pornographic images (advertising) would flash on the screen and she would immediately turn them off. But children inside her had seen them. Little children who had been used in pornographic films. They saw the images, and saw she was looking for films, and thought they were about to be abused again. So they made her drink alcohol, because her main abuser had fed her alcohol to make her compliant while she was posed for the pictures. The alcohol made the filming bearable. Fifty years later, they were preparing for abuse that was never going to happen again. I explained to them that they were safe now, and then I explained to the adult front person what was triggering her drinking. She was very relieved that she was not an addict or an alcoholic after all, and she agreed not to surf on any websites she did not already know were entirely safe. She could have figured this out for herself if she had simply asked inside; she did not need me to do that for her.

If you are a survivor of organized abuse, and you start to develop anxiety, or overreactions, or an addiction, there is one important thing you can do: Ask inside. Ask your insiders, especially the children, what is bothering them. What mistaken beliefs or feelings, based on memories from the past, are causing the symptoms? Unless the cause is current abuse, you will be able to solve the problem by working together with your inside children. If the cause is current abuse, however, you have a more serious problem, but it is better to face up to it than to remain ignorant of it and continue to be abused without awareness. If it is current abuse, you need to work on a way to make it stop or to escape.

If you are a therapist, when you see symptoms in a dissociative person, it is important to focus on the person's internal dynamics rather than on the known external events of present-day life. For example, you might ask:

"May I speak with your insiders to find out whether something is bothering them?"

Front people often resist this: "No, it's just me, I've got plenty of problems." They are afraid of finding yet another terrifying memory that they would prefer not to learn about. You could respond:

"Inside kids often have reactions to things in your life, and their feelings may leak through to you. Just let me check, or maybe you'd rather ask them yourself."

Then you, or the client, checks with the insiders and the explanation is often pretty straightforward.

Asking inside is very important for all survivors, not just for solving problems like these but for managing daily life and for resolving your traumas. If you are a survivor, in order to heal well, you need to meet your insiders' needs. You can do this best if you ask them what they need. If you have a flashback or a nightmare, it is probably coming from some inner part who is stuck in that memory and does not know how things have changed. Your internal leaders can find that part and rescue him or her, update that part on present life and safety (if you are safe), and put that memory on the waiting list for processing. If you have physical pain, you can ask your insiders whether someone inside is in pain from a memory, or whether someone has been recently hurt, or whether the body is actually ill. You cannot figure these things out without talking with your insiders. This is why the perpetrators forbid your front person to communicate internally. This is why you must do what they do not want you to do.

Mind-controlled and frozen in time

Wendy Hoffman

Many survivors feel that the after effects of traumatic abuse dominate their lives. The majority of each survivor's life is spent in ordinary life, usually handled by the front person with relatively ordinary thoughts and feelings. Still, there are always dark flashes and strange sensations leaking from survivors' depths, especially if something in ordinary life happens to touch on what really happened.

Satanic rituals occur at most once a month normally. That is three to four hours taken up per month. Programming sessions take place during childhood once a week while the programmers are splitting the brain and inserting commands that they consider to be lifelong and that they want followed. Maintenance programming occurs far less frequently. Punishment tortures usually occur no more than once a month. Some groups just hold rituals seasonally. Some master-madmen like Mengele and Cameron hold all-night mind-control sessions, but those are rare. So, the actual time spent being tortured and/or mind-controlled is a small fraction of the total time you spend in ordinary life doing everyday actions. Yet, the impact of the monthly ritual and weekly mind-control session is almost constant in your life.

The terror does not get a chance to subside. At times, during ordinary life, you may not feel the terror, but it is there all the time, sizzling like a volcano waiting to erupt. Parts inside you experience heightened terror constantly.

There is more than a residue of powerlessness and defeat. Those feelings make up the backbone of the survivors' lives and do not easily abate. The anxiety is strong enough to move a mountain.

When non-traumatic events occur, they wash away in time and eventually are not recalled. But traumatic occurrences stick and freeze out the cleansing flow of time. They become cemented and cannot be budged or prodded out. They took up such a relatively small amount of time, yet consistently control the personalities and mind-set. They form your cognitions about life and prevent entering life fully. They wash over many of life's other experiences and form the negative self-concept.

Cult groups must feel quite threatened lately. If they are worried about one of their victims, they might hold torture sessions nightly. That is one of their innovations. It may hurt but not be more effective. Nightly sessions are usually held if the victim is under a form of house arrest, such as living in a perpetrator's home as a guest or prisoner, or with a roommate, parent, sibling, or child who is a trained perpetrator and torturer.

The mind-control designers knew the principle of the younger you are, the more intensely you feel. The rigidity and endurance of these emotions and beliefs go back to infancy, as do new programs and commands. The new ones are rooted in earlier programming that took place in infancy and childhood.

If the traumas of rituals and mind control have such potent and lasting impact, is there any way to lessen their blow? Can, for example, a smiley face become just the common smiley face and not a trigger to report back to a handler? Or can a playing card, say the Jack of clubs or spades flashed at you, not be read as a trigger to kill yourself or someone else? Can objects of day-to-day life lose their associations and become simply what they are and not loaded with perverse meaning?

If the front person and other parts do not know what the rest of the system has experienced and endured, the feelings from the traumatic life will remain alive though buried. As the system unearths what is held inside and understands how all those feelings and wounds got there, they will have the opportunity to be released and healed. But they have to be remembered and re-experienced, though very briefly. If they remain unknown and hidden, they will stay alive and untouched, unfortunately.

If the front person has become co-conscious or integrated with the rest of the system, those feelings and cognitions will begin their healing journey on their own. Inside parts are not oblivious. They can perceive when life has changed, when they are no longer victims, when they can touch freedom. How you feel behind bars and how you feel in a grassy meadow are different. The insiders will realize there is no reason to bring a barred prison onto a field of wild flowers. Reality can catch up with tortured insiders.

Even after you are free from the tortured intensity of keeping the trauma alive, even after you have accomplished considerable repairing of yourself, you might not feel the way other people feel. Why should you? Your life has not been like theirs and even if they want to try, they can never conceive of what your experiences were like. They can imagine the heart of evil but they do not know it. Some people will be kind to you, but you may still feel lonely. The loneliness will not have the intensity you used to feel because you are no longer composed of many tortured infants and children, some of whom lost the only person they thought loved them. You will probably spend time nurturing yourself. You have been through a great deal. Now is the time to go slowly, to rock yourself, to care for the chronic physical injuries, to step away from intensity and frozenness, to soothe and love yourself for who you have been and who you are. If the infant pieces inside you still need healing, sing lullabies to them.

It would be lovely to say that relationships will be good from now on and that life is sweet. But that is not realistic. Sometimes it is depressing for survivors to be with normal people, even kind ones. Many of them are relaxed within themselves and their bodies, love life, and have many pleasant memories that make up their being. They are even relaxed about their mistakes. They do not think they have to be perfect. And they have family relationships that have buoyed them up, even if they occasionally tear them down. Survivors, even healed ones, have strips of ice and rage within. They grew up under such intense conditions that normal recreational activities do not usually do it for them. They rarely have nurturing memories to fall back on and often prefer to be alone. Whoever you are, you are. Praise yourself for being you. Believe in yourself.

The strong and brave ones (previously known as the garbage kids)

Alison Miller

I have known for a long time that that many survivors of mind control and ritual abuse have insider parts called the garbage kids or expendables (or, in the UK, rubbish kids). They are to be found, naked and dirty and smelling of urine, in internal garbage dumps, usually with nasty things like insects and rotting flesh. These places in the inner world are copies of real-world places where these parts were dumped when they violated the abusers' rules by refusing to obey important commands. Several times I have assisted survivor clients in rescuing the garbage kids, cleaning them up, and giving them clothes and comfortable, warm internal places to live. But until recently I have not thought about the strengths of these insiders or the ways in which they can help with recovery.

Recently, a client's young insiders were telling me about a group of internal girls trapped under the floorboards of the internal copy of the primary abuser's living room, put there as a punishment for disobedience. I searched for insiders who were brave enough to get them out of the room where the internal copy of the abuser was asleep in a chair. The ones I was talking with said, "I'm not brave," "I'm weak," "She might catch me." I realized I needed some insiders who were strong and brave, and I thought of the garbage kids, who had been rescued (by self-created parts who lived in the trees) from an outdoor garbage dump. Like the girls under the boards, they were courageous and outspoken. We planned to ask the garbage kids to go where the obedient ones had not dared to go.

Another survivor client has been struggling with a bullying supervisor at work (in the real world). This boss intimidates her by micromanaging her work, and saying things like "Are you all right?" This brings out (just behind the front person) the little girls who feel afraid of bullies like their father, and the adult feels anxious and close to tears, although previously she was feeling all right.

The first thing we tried was enlisting the top soldiers in her now cooperative system to strengthen the front person. We were both surprised that this did not work, and we had to figure out why. These "tough guys" were actually, like anyone in the military, trained to obey orders instantly rather than to defy authority. They (or rather, the discarded parts from whom they had been split off) had been severely punished for any assertiveness or sign of insubordination. These seemingly strong leaders were, therefore, very vulnerable to the bullying supervisor, trying much too hard to follow orders even when the orders made no sense. Although they had given orders in the inside world, they had always obeyed in the outside world, and even though they did not show their emotions, they were dominated by fear.

So, we thought hard about who should be present with the adult front person in the workplace. And we thought of the garbage kids. These were the ones who had stood up to authority despite the punishment. They were willing to be assertive—which was exactly what was needed. They accompanied the adult to work for the next week. She found herself able to stand up to her supervisor, make a good argument when the supervisor was wrong, and resist intimidation. The supervisor's bullying decreased as she realized the survivor was not going to react the way she wanted her to.

Find your garbage kids, and make good use of their strengths when you need the courage to stand up for yourself or what you believe is right.

Survivors and illness

Wendy Hoffman

Like everyone else in the world, survivors get sick. They get sick because of germs or viruses or diseases like cancer, or as reactions to their having been abused and tortured, or some combination of both.

When survivors become ill, they have to deal with the symptoms of the illness and all that these symptoms evoke. Body memories can creep into the experience of sickness. The body memories can derive from what happened a long time ago. The brain experiences what was done in the far distance as if it were happening in the present time. Survivors are, and have been, fairly regularly tortured. In their everyday life, they probably do not know about the physical abuses; otherwise they would immediately leave their areas and go into hiding. They stay because their parts who live ordinary lives do not know that the night before they were tortured almost to death.

When survivors have serious illnesses with agonizing symptoms, unconscious memories of the torture scenes may emerge. The real pain waltzes with the remembered pain and the agony becomes magnified. Unless the other parts of the brain are integrated with their front parts, the ill survivors will not know they are dealing with a mixture of real and recalled symptoms. One survivor's intestinal infection awoke parts who had always felt that way when they had been starved and purged in preparation for a ritual. Her parts turned on the "keep awake" program (made by poking her whenever she fell asleep) because they thought a ritual was imminent. This went on for weeks, and as a result her recovery from the illness was delayed.

Here are some danger spots for the sick survivor: If the memories start to become more real in a survivor's conscious knowing, she might temporarily lose her will to live. In the middle of fighting a real illness, this development can be fatal.

Another complication is survivors' hypersensitivity to chemical drugs. At least when I was an infant, perpetrators used to place babies on sheets doused in chemicals, to increase their misery and make sure they felt abandoned. Over the years, other, stronger chemicals are used to sedate or control them. Eventually, the victims may develop an intolerance to any kind of chemicals. The medicines doctors prescribe often produce rashes and other dangerous side effects.

Most doctors will not believe survivors' pasts so it may not pay to tell them.

Some survivors might do better with holistic doctors. They can take the holistic medicine and not react to chemicals. Holistic doctors probably will not believe the stories either.

When survivors become ill, there is a potential for complications. Be armed with good self-care, a comfortable bed, lots of juices in the fridge, chicken soup in the freezer just in case, and the knowledge that you may have to fight to have a will to live. Do not do memory work until you are well, even though body memories are present. Put the narrative on hold for a while.

If you have support people in your life, allow them to help and comfort you. This is a time when you need help no matter how independent you may want to be and are.

However, this is when family usually moves in, even if you have separated from them and attempted to cut off contact. They are always looking for a way to get back in your life. Local informants and spies may tell them you are ill and vulnerable at present. This is a moment they might regain control of you, all in the guise of wanting to help their own. They will be destroying you as they look good to the world.

If possible, do not let handlers, programmers, informants, or "friends" know that you are ill or injured. If they find out, they will most likely use this time to insert other program and torture sessions into your life. They take advantage of weaknesses. They prey on vulnerabilities. They will use vulnerabilities that occur by chance and those that they create. Imitate animal behavior and hide the pain and weakness from them.

For example, when I was stung by an underground hive of yellow jackets and had an allergic reaction, my torturer immediately wanted to visit. I had not had contact with her for months prior to this mishap. At that time, I did not know she was a programmer and torturer and had been assigned to me. She is not a generous or helpful person, but she wanted access to my house. I told her I was too sick for company. She offered to stay in a motel and just visit with her husband for a few minutes. Fortunately, I said no. However, because I was ill, I could have used someone who was genuinely helpful to look after me.

If you do not have honest support people in your life, and you need help with basic activities like bringing in groceries, cooking, or walking your dog, consider hiring a home health aide. Be careful about where you get the recommendations from. An agency's referrals may be safer. I got a referral from a "friend" who turned out to be the leader of a coven where I live. I did not know that at the time. This particular home health aide was safe and good. Still, it is better to be cautious.

Medical doctors have tortured victims of these mind-control abuses. People with intelligence and medical abilities who are born into these groups are spotted through aptitude tests, sent to medical school, and become the cult doctors who torture and program. In the church I had been forced to attend, the cult-involved leaders sent a young lawyer to medical school, because they needed the services of a lawyer–doctor. Because of past abuse by doctors, victims are usually afraid of physicians and avoid medical treatment even when they need it. Sometimes, they delay treatment for too long. Most medical professionals are not cult people. Use your inner sense and judgment when attempting to find an honest doctor. Do not get a referral from anyone who might be cult involved.

Hospitals might present an even greater threat to recovery. Most of us were abused in hospitals at some time in our lives. Some hospitals have been taken over by cult personnel, others only partly. Some hospitals are clean and honest. When I lay semi-unconscious in a rural Delaware hospital recovering from a long-delayed surgery, my ex-boyfriend/handler entered with a woman who looked like me. Perhaps they thought I would be jealous of her, but I pitied her. These two had planned to murder me by placing poisons in the IV. He tortured me before she heard the nurse's footsteps coming down the hall that warned him. They fled uncaught. That is routine practice. It is no wonder we survivors avoid hospitals. Nonetheless, there are some safe ones and times when a hospital can save your life.

If/when you get a serious illness, stop all extraneous activity, even recovery work, and focus solely on self-care and becoming well again. Be careful of who surrounds you.

Life in the midst of cultists is hard enough when you are well and healthy. Reserve the tiny bit of strength you may have for keeping your illness secret from the enemy. Because your whole life is a war zone, you are equipped to handle the danger. Your life has been a rehearsal for recovering from illness.

Things will not last forever

Wendy Hoffman

I used to think that all bad or unpleasant things would last forever. This false belief filled me with chronic dread. If I had to go to a film I did not want to watch, I felt the experience would never end. At a noisy restaurant, the bad meal would be everlasting. Visits with people I did not like might never stop. Family vacations. Lectures. Anxiety and guilt could be constants. Physical pain, never ending.

After I achieved considerable recovery, when the belief in frozen ever-afterness evaporated, I had to consider why I had felt like that before.

Programmers create personalities that they say live in isolated containers. They teach the victims' minds to believe that lie, and they show a physical representation of the prison-containers to the child victims. Children do not know these parts and pieces were splintered off from the main brain, the mainland, through drugs, torture, isolation, and lies. They do not consciously know with their whole minds that these segregated parts have been made to falsely believe that they live in boxes, wells, freezers, caves, tubes, tunnels, cages, or other such holding containers. Sadistic programmers split off these parts when the body was young. Having no further life experience, these parts remain at that age for the rest of the body's lifespan or until they break out or are rescued. In the beginning of recovery, few personalities can become aware of themselves without outside help.

Many parts of the brain are frozen indefinitely. These sections live in a stasis. Consequently, the whole system absorbs the feeling of any one state becoming permanent, without interruption, without relief. Hence, the dread of life.

After recovery, one of the previously persistent attitudes that disappears is this boxed-in feeling that things last forever. As the barricades imposed on the mind fall away, the boxes and other containers open, personalities are released from their prisons, and attitudes naturally alter enormously. The brain parts realize they had been separated and imprisoned against their will. Released, they do fast growing and catching up and experience a multitude of emotions. They gradually mature from where they started, which may be younger than five, to the biological body's age. Consequently, this feeling of entrapment and the unpleasant sensation of stasis fall away.

In reality, things do not last forever. Balance replaces this dread. Dinners end. So do films, conversations, and relationships. Everything is in flux, just as the ancient Lucretius claimed. Like rivers, with highs and lows, floods and droughts, and balance. One summer, you cannot water your lawn. That fall, the rivers overflow. To see things as stasis is not to see reality. Even electroshock ends. And ignorance. And mind control. And torture.

You can be with people you do not particularly like and know it will end in an hour or two. You can endure a bad meal in a noisy restaurant for an hour and a half. Feelings pass. Some are unpleasant or even torturing, but they do not last a lifetime. Everything is fluid, always changing. Some emotions and relationships endure because you want them to, not because they seem inescapable. One sign of healing is knowing that lids have been raised and time is not stuck.

Even before recovery, beauty can impose relief to this unfortunate, bursting intensity. To be close to nature, feel the earth with your feet, see snow-covered mountains, and oceans. All this natural beauty can help dissolve the steel barriers between personalities and release the lids of their containers. Becoming whole is a life-long process that the experience of beauty encourages. Even in ugly, dirty, noisy cities, there are spots of beauty. I used to live in Manhattan. I walked to a park on the upper Westside and sat near its colorful, fragrant garden. I am sure that reprieve from the hardness of my life aided my memory process.

Rushed

Wendy Hoffman

I was late for my friend's New Year's lunch. My dog was taking too long outside and I only half remembered my friend's address. I began rushing. There was something about that rushed feeling that was startling and familiar.

I remembered. My legal father had what they now call poor impulse control. He seemed incapable of waiting for anything. He would rush my mother brutally if he wanted the family to go somewhere. Instead of helping in the house, he stood at the front door screaming, which seemed to make her go more slowly. Or if a car ahead of him went more slowly than he wanted, this father cursed loudly and called other drivers "one-eyed monkeys."

But there was worse—so much worse. Mind control is time-limited. You can only keep children in electroshock chairs for a finite amount of time. If the electroshocks are unlimited, children can die. If they die, what is the sense of mind controlling them? There's a feeling of pressure and impatience during mind control sessions:

- Deliver up a new piece of your mind to hold this program.
- Learn the cue.
- Memorize the trigger.

- We do not have all day.
- Hidden electroshock chairs are in high demand. Multitudes of unfortunate children need programming. They all need turns in the chairs. Hurry up and get programmed.
- Time is money.

It often takes a team to program one individual.

The faster the better. Going too slowly ups the intensity of the torture.

Even if these attitudes are not verbalized, they are felt. Victims feel them.

Victims have to give over possession of their minds and souls, and they have to do it quickly or else.

Another danger inherent in programming sessions is that programmers, even master ones or perhaps especially the master ones, can turn psychotic in a flash. If they become psychotic while working on a child, they can up the torture unbearably, maim, or murder the victim child. It is best for the children to finish the programming session as quickly as possible. And at the end, they sometimes get a treat. A tootsie roll in exchange for a brain.

When I felt rushed this afternoon, I thought of my legal father and the even more pernicious programming sessions—the bullying, sinister rushing and being forced to give up my mind. *My* mind.

I do puzzles online. The computer times how long you take to solve the jigsaw puzzle. I will not hurry. I will not be rushed. I do not care how long I take. It is not a race for me. Never again.

Mind control cults with high international aspirations test their child victims all the time. They give them multiple-choice questions. Time is one factor in how they are judged. They have to answer columns of questions as quickly as possible. They have to beat the other contestants, who might have been their friends. They have to go faster and faster.

Never again.

Then I remembered how impatient I used to be. If we were supposed to leave at a certain time, I had trouble waiting for dawdlers. I was impatient with people slow to catch on. That kind of icy impatience is programmed into certain cult roles. I became like the queen playing croquet in *Alice in Wonderland,* cold and bitchy. As I left these roles, I at last shed this imposed impatience and became more human.

SECTION VII
THE HEALING PROCESS

How to begin to console the inconsolable

Wendy Hoffman

There are not enough therapists to treat all the survivors who want to come out of slavery and who are screaming for help. Most therapists do not have a clue about what mind control entails. Some are afraid. Some of their partners, spouses, and children are too fearful. Many do not have the curiosity or the intelligence to read everything and educate themselves. Some do not want to learn by trial and error. Consequently, there is a dearth of competent therapists for this field.

So, except for the lucky few, we will have to find another way.

Alison wrote an excellent step-by-step guide to treating yourselves in the absence of a professional in her book, *Becoming Yourself* (2014).

Here are the two drawbacks among many to guard against as you plow through the morass of mind control on your own or even with a therapist:

1. Be aware all the time that you have been deceived. Question everything. Do not assume that because you think it, it is true. Your mind from infancy on has been filled with distortions and fantasy. Refine your sense of logic to help you ascertain what is real and what is yet another lie they fed you.

2. The most serious problem is that intense feelings of isolation will emerge as you work through your mind control and torture. When you were a baby and all alone in a family that was not allowed to love and had to hate, you lost your sense of attachment. You might have clung desperately to the desire to have a consoling adult caregiver but the script for children born into solid cult families is that there cannot be attachments and bonding.

These intense feelings of isolation and aloneness will be present throughout your self-recovery. Some of you will have the incredibly good luck to have found a partner or spouse who cares and knows how to listen. I wish we all had that kind of luck. We deserve it. Even a part-time friend could help. A therapist is often a part-time friend. Do not count on anyone else in the family seeking freedom, though it can occasionally happen.

You have to find a way to relieve these intense feelings of devastation even if you end up again alone with them. You need an internal system to help alleviate the intensity.

Perhaps some empathetic, loving inner parts could come forward to mother, rock, nurture, and feed. These feelings will usually reside in infants with no understanding of why adults act cruelly. Hold these infants' hearts in your motherly hands, tell them that they are good babies, that they are not to blame. The infants and small children cannot understand the concept of lying and deceit. Their minds cannot yet take in abstractions.

If you are loved, you feel lovable. If you are despised and rejected and tortured, you feel like a rag.

Love these inner infants who hold your desolation. You are lovable. They are lovable.

Online support groups can help break some of the isolation, but these feelings of aloneness are often too intense even to put into words.

If you do not see the same benign people at work or school every week, try to join a weekly in-person group and sit with the familiar people. The group does not have to be a mind control and ritual abuse recovery group. In fact, it is probably safer if it is not. Its regularity can interrupt isolation.

If you have a pet, stay close to that animal. Feel its pulse of life in your hands. That should help.

Eat the comfort food you need, unless you have a medical condition that says you should not. In general, this is not the time to worry about your weight.

Once you integrate, the whole system can hold the devastation of loneliness and its intensity will lessen. Each part in you has to release the treacherous feelings. Then, as the intensity lessens, you will want to isolate less. The rest of your life does not have to be spent in this aloneness. Even if you live for only a few more years, it is worth doing the work and getting a taste of what life was designed to be. If you are pursued and still not safe, it is better to isolate yourself until you are 100% sure someone is safe.

These most devastating feelings are usually found underneath rage. First, infants are angry, then sad. Unless we work hard to find these infant experiences, we may remain trapped in them. Even people who were never abused have this pattern of falling back on young emotions. At any age, it is wise to find all of yourself.

The body remembers

Wendy Hoffman

If you are dissociative and know it because someone you trust told you, how do you get back to remembering what happened to make you that way?

Catch the flashes of reality that intrude into your consciousness while you do mindless activities; do spontaneous art work that does not care about technique; hold onto your dreams and work on understanding them, especially nightmares; listen to your body. It talks. It informs you. It knows. If you lived with family more violent than conniving killer dogs, your body will have that information. The body has a direct route to the brain. The brain can open and tell. It can overcome its capture.

Have you chronic pain? Suppose your left arm aches from time to time, not always. If you concentrate your energy on that arm and ask the many parts inside you who know about this pain, some might come out and tell. Try to gather everyone together who knows something about this ache, if it is possible. This one body ailment can open the door to a universe of memory. You may be, in your memory process, plunged into a ritual site, see an altar. You may be holding a sacrificial sword. Someone robed may be forcing you to murder. If you have a memory like this, it will be one among many. But you are there, in the middle of this scene. It would not have opened had you not wanted it to and been ready. It can never be pleasant. It is the road to freedom—freedom that you never had but craved.

Some survivors may have noticed that their head shakes periodically for no apparent reason. It just bobs up and down on your neck as if controlled by an outside force. In some instances, there is no medical explanation for this phenomenon. It is memories of electroshock. If survivors can follow their jerking heads to their root cause, being shocked with electricity probably throughout their lives to date, they will find themselves in the heart of mind control. Once they have memories of being stripped naked and a helmet placed on them, strapped into electroshock chairs, drugged, then they can recapture the commands and programs that until now have ruled their lives. The body can lead the closed-down mind to a chance at life.

I had black and blue marks of various sizes along my spine. The largest was the size of a tablespoon, the smallest a teaspoon. During a massage in the 1990s, a physical therapist asked what had caused them. I told this hardworking, innocent Swiss woman they were from needles going into my vertebrae during mind control procedures from infancy on. She had asked and I told. She became so panicky that she went for supervision. Unfortunately, her supervisor was a cult plant. There went my confidentiality, right out the window. Over two decades later, I finally found a safe, knowledgeable, tough therapist. I told Alison about my bad experience with the physical therapist and wanted to show her my bruised back. I lifted my shirt.

"They're not there," she said with a flat voice.

"Yes, they are," I said and pointed insistently to where they once were last time I looked, maybe last year.

"They're not there," she said. I rushed to the bathroom mirror and strained my neck to turn. I did not see them either. "They vanished. Why? I had them for seventy years."

"Because they're not needed anymore. You already remembered."

Do not ever underestimate the power of the brain and its marionette, the body. The body will shoot up physical pain, it will knock hard and repeatedly against your conscious awareness until you acknowledge it. When you get to the facts it conveys, when you work it through and out, it will leave you and take with it all the breadcrumbs it has left in its path to your knowledge. You will then have peace in this particular area. If weeks, months, or years later, the pain or marks or emotions return, it means there is more to the memory, another piece to work through and dissolve. Recovery requires endurance.

A question that haunts most survivors in recovery is how to tell the difference between a body memory and a real medical illness. In general, body memories come and go and medical illnesses are steady. However, some medical illnesses assert and withdraw and are not constant. Toothaches can be inconstant, earaches, stomachaches, even headaches. So constancy is not an infallible determination. Time sometimes tells. If you focus on what is underneath a pain, often the answer becomes clear. Or you can get a check-up from your doctor, if that is not too traumatic. Sensitivity to your body, which allows it to defrost, and willingness to follow the pain wherever it leads, will often take you to the doorstep of truth.

Bodily pain can also indicate recent abuse. If the doctors are not finding an illness, and your inside parts are not coming up with memories to match the pain, you might need to look for hidden parts who hold the awareness of current harassment and abuse.

Flashbacks also torment people. Those who suffer from PTSD symptoms can befriend their haunting flashbacks, which follow them like a hired detective, and make a pact with them. They can be reconsidered and thought of as a road to knowledge. Thank you, flashbacks, for making me deal with this. They are like panic attacks and body memories, not arbitrary, not from nowhere. They come as direct messengers to tell you what happened to you and what is not yet consciously known or resolved. They are the key to the lost selves. Go after them.

Ten keys to recovery*

Alison Miller

1. Acknowledge your multiplicity. Mind control is entirely based on splitting the mind in infancy. All survivors have inner parts who were trained, whether or not they are aware of these parts.
2. Communicate internally. Think to your insiders and listen to their responses. Insiders, talk to one another to discover how each of you was deceived.
3. The inner parts the abusers placed in charge of the personality system need to take the lead in working towards recovery, along with any self-created strong parts. Let the front person manage everyday life while the rest of the system works on recovery.
4. Improve your inner world. Get children out of the internal copies of places where they were abused. Give insiders new jobs to replace their old ones. Make sure your internal government cares for the needs of all parts.
5. Recovery begins with finding a way to become physically safe. Dismantle your access programming: the training to report to abusers, return to them, and come when they call you.

* This chapter was presented at the 2015 *Survivorship* Conference, and is in the online journal *Survivorship*, Fall 2015.

6. All programming is based on the BIG LIE, which is that the abusers know where you are and what you say and/or think at all times. Let your whole personality system know that the BIG LIE is a lie. The abusers only know what you do or say or think if your reporter parts tell them or if someone you know tells on you.
7. Choose a safe therapist. Willingness to learn may be more important in a therapist than knowledge.
8. Once you are safe enough, you can begin the memory work which thoroughly undoes the programming.
9. You can choose whether to work through all your traumatic memories, or just achieve stability. Which you choose may depend on your age and health and present-day real-world responsibilities. Closed down and stable are not the same as healed; closed down people have hidden hurt children inside. But full healing takes a long time and works best with a skilled therapist.
10. Integration and co-consciousness come naturally as a result of memory work; do not focus on them. Allow inside parts to join as they are ready.

The nobility of survivors

Wendy Hoffman

There are levels of being in survivors, all put in by their enemies. First, their perpetrators empty them out so that they become distant from who they are. Programmers build an amnesic wall around the original self in an attempt to make the self's disappearance permanent. Then they layer in the many functions they want their newly created commodity to perform. They may create, for example, an assassin, mule, prostitute, pornography star, breeder, thief, soldier, cult therapist, and so on.

Eventually, nowadays, some survivors gravitate to therapy to try to find out who they really are and what their lives have contained. Some are fortunate enough to end up with safe therapists not employed and trained by the groups they are attempting to escape. Those receive help.

Some of the professional experts in the field are also writers and write about their clients' experiences and personalities. They describe children used in pedophiles' parties, their clients' rage, broken lives, being institutionalized. They describe lives directed by others' commands where survivors become like ping-pong balls—battered here, sent here, sent there, told to do this—all without a will of their own.

What is sometimes, not always, missed is why some survivors agree to be mindless in the first place. Yes, there are amnesic barriers preventing them from knowing what they are being forced to do and what they never consciously would do. But there must be something else.

Not all, but many, therapist–writers miss the original threat and decision. What is it originally that makes it almost impossible to escape?

Ironically, it is integrity. Integrity leads one into the most dismal of lives.

For instance, perpetrators tell their victims that someone they love will be murdered or have a limb or limbs amputated unless they comply. The children with compassion are willing to sacrifice themselves to save others. Survivors are not just marionettes performing criminal secret functions. They are also self-sacrificing heroes trying to protect others. The people they attempt to save might have even been cruel and destructive to them. Perpetrators tell children that a universal bomb will go off unless they follow hideous orders. They said that even before the age of terrorism. And it is not all about nepotism. Survivors still thinking as children also attempt to protect strangers. They care about a world that has abandoned them.

Where does this charitable sweetness come from? Children are innocent, think they cause everything to happen, want power, importance, and recognition, and for everything to be nice and safe. Adult survivors have children inside, frozen in their ages and development.

It is unlikely that perpetrator threats would be carried out. If they were, these secret cults would be eliminating so many people, there would have to be investigations and common knowledge. That is the last thing they want. The legal and police forces could never accommodate such massive investigations. Moreover, the people they are threatening to murder are often the people they think they own, the people they control and have invested effort and money in creating. They are not necessarily the people they want eliminated. Perpetrators depend on their victims remaining in states of immature thinking so that they cannot think things through realistically.

When working with survivors, as a professional or a support person, or simply as someone who cares, it is important to dig deeper into the original decisions and choices. The excavations have to go into the areas of the original selves where the heart of the child lives. They say children are cruel, but not these children. They do not start out that way. These children know compassion and self-sacrifice. They care about others even more than they care about themselves. Although they have never been protected, they protect others.

One advantage of living into adulthood is that you get the opportunity to think in life as an adult and not stay trapped in child-think. Some are able to break free of that limited capacity. Usually with help, their minds can catch up with their biological age.

As adults, you can reverse the choices of childhood. Even as you rethink early and unconscious decisions, you become aware of the integrity of your early responses. You have to respect yourself for that.

The investigations into lost selves have to plow down deeper into the inherent nobility of survivors' choices. It is unfortunate that nobility leads survivors into destruction. As adults, however, all that can be reversed while integrity and nobility are maintained. Look at the integrity working through these layers of imposed deceit requires.

How many people sacrifice their own lives to protect someone else? Yes, it was all most likely a response to a lie, but children have no way of knowing that. Only in adulthood can you figure it out. How many people care so much about other human beings as children do?

After integration, the naïve sweetness of the child mind dissolves and you become more self-protective. The new nobility becomes understanding the awful ordering of your inside parts and acknowledges yourself. You realize that it does not pay to sacrifice yourself for people commissioned to destroy you, even if this commission is against their will.

Self-esteem loosens mind control*

Wendy Hoffman

People who have had fairly normal lives do not know the kinds of emotions survivors experience. The intensity of these feelings separates us with the most dense barricade from normal people, that is, those who have not been mind-controlled and who have not attended homicidal rituals. The human being was not built to sustain such feelings, and these feelings have associated strong false beliefs about ourselves.

Here are some examples of the kinds of beliefs and associated feelings I am addressing.

- Guilt: I am responsible for babies' and children's deaths.
- I am worthless, stupid, ugly, taking up room on earth for nothing but myself.
- I am a blight on the earth. My evil spreads everywhere and contaminates and infects everyone.
- I am nothing. It is my fault that . . .

* A version of this essay was presented at the Survivorship Ritual Abuse and Child Abuse 2016 Conference "Stop Mind Control and Programs", in Oakland, CA.

- I must be bad or my mother (or father) would love me.
- If I ever make a mistake, it proves that I am a bad person.
- I am ashamed of myself. I feel flooded with shame.

Along with these feelings are orders about the world and mind-controlled behaviors programmed into us by the cult, such as:

- You are not allowed to bond.
- You belong to us [meaning to your programmers and family].
- Do not run—you cannot run away from us and your programmers.
- We will find you wherever you go.
- You will never be free.
- We know what you think and say, etc.
- Everyone will always hate you; you will never have friends.
- You are so different that you will never fit in, you will always be an outcast.

Your controllers employ all the above lies and others, as well as these kinds of twisted statements to make you feel bad about yourself:

- We had to kill him or her because you loved him or her.
- Your mother is unhappy because you are ugly. (Then they will program the mother to be depressed and perhaps stay in bed all day.)
- You have to be a sex slave because you are not good for anything else.
- One parent at best will not love you.
- You are stupid, that is why you cannot learn in school. (Programmers put in the learning disabilities.)
- If you were good, your mother would love you. Your mother loves your brother or sister.

Survivors go into therapy expecting to find out horrible things about themselves. They are sure on some deep level that they are bad, evil people. That is what they have been taught from earliest childhood. An effective way of loosening this mind control is to more accurately access who you are in reality.

Re-evaluating yourself is crucial. You have to learn to love yourself. You have to be committed to such unlearning and learning. We were taught we were bad, to blame, that we wanted crime and evil, that we were ugly and loathsome. All those statements are lies. As you process your memories, possibly in therapy, you will see how you were controlled and forced to do what they make you do.

You are not an evil witch or wizard. You are an innocent victim. You will discover actions and feelings that you are not proud of, but you did not start out evil. You were forced and coerced into doing what they wanted you to do, for their own gain, not yours. Recovery allows you to break free of that mold. We all regret what was done to us and what we consequently became. But now is the time to change all that. Now is the time to become your self. It is time to ask "Who am I?" without the mind control.

Who are you?

The two bad things that dent even normal people's minds and souls are rejection and abandonment. The first thing perpetrators do for some is create abandonment while you are still in the womb. Once born, abandonment and rejection are practiced routinely. Abuse and group abuse occur throughout childhood. Parents deliver and abandon the child. This emotional terrain makes mind control and programming easy for the perpetrators. They want to make you feel like a nothing. They need that horrible or non-existent self-esteem for the mind control to work.

Also, the mind has to be young and vulnerable. As soon as it forms into a cohesive whole, programs are much harder to put in. Even torture cannot put them in. That is why these cults maintain members in every generation. You have to give over your children because they need them to learn to do their assigned criminal acts and be robots. Can you call mindless robots who have no memory or judgment criminals? Mind control festers within children who have been abandoned and rejected.

Nothing is more crucial than, or a substitute for, working through the programs and hierarchy of inside parts and the braiding and offshoots of parts. But if you work through all that mind control but not on the emotional terrain and the concept of self-esteem, you end up like a dry drunk. You have overcome the addiction but not developed as a full human being. You have not then caught up with the life that was taken from you. The self-esteem piece comes in before, during, and after the hard main work of working through the mind control. The self-esteem piece entails thinking boldly. It is not easy to break through amnesic barriers, but it is a pleasure to see them dissolve.

Moreover, whether you can work your way through a complicated maze of dissociation depends on your self-esteem. As different sequestered parts in you begin to speak and you begin finally to listen, you will hear strange things coming out of your mouth.

The question is whether to believe. Where is the information coming from? Is it coming directly from a part created through mind control? Ask whether the part is repeating what it is supposed to say. Tell that part it no longer has to do that. If it is not repeating, you might want to believe what that part says, no matter how unpleasant and contrary to the image of your front person.

Whether you can believe what is not programmed and comes out of your mouth depends on your belief in yourself—on your self-esteem. It depends on your commitment to healing yourself. So many survivors spend a great deal of therapy time—years and decades—deliberating whether or not to believe their insiders.

Sometimes, parts will have wrong ideas or lies that controllers placed in them. When you and the parts and pieces of you finally communicate, you can help them see that they have been living under the impact of untruths. Examples would be that the programmers and handlers can hear and know everything they think and say, that they have to tell if they change addresses, that someone they love will be killed if they disobey. When you bump into one of these programs, it is an opportunity to trace it to its origin. Follow the thread of parts to the training session where a new piece of you was created and given instructions on how to behave, act, think, believe, and forget. Every lie you discover that you have believed is an opportunity to delve into how they molded you.

If you want freedom to be who you are, it is crucial to listen to the insiders who alone know what your life has been. Each insider has a piece of reality. All the pieces have to be put together if you want full healing. You have to find the hidden pieces, the parts the programmers hid so that a full healing could never take place. But you can find them. Inside parts will lead you to their hiding places. Or they will be uncovered in time as other parts that hid them move away and their hiding places are exposed. From the outside or front person, you cannot figure out your life. You have to listen to those who experienced it. Whether to believe what they say depends on the strength of your belief in yourself.

At first, my insiders would not talk to me. I was already sixty-nine years old. I started writing to them and they wrote back. A short time later, they began to form words in my head and I could say or think words back to them. Then I asked questions and they answered. I could hardly believe the answers, but my recovery had begun. It all depended on the communication between the outside and inside me's. I remember the first time I spoke with Alison on the phone from opposite sides of two countries. She asked my insiders questions. They did not answer and the rest of me did not know. She asked again in another way. No answer or "I do not know." And again. She suggested I write down an answer. They wrote using my hand. Then I wrote questions. They wrote answers. As the days went on, we began to talk to one another and, awake and asleep, we began to think to one another. This dialogue is essential if you want to get to know your insiders. Your outside is important for reaching in and, of course, for keeping your ordinary life going. Can you imagine—most people in the world only have to deal with ordinary life. But not us. For us, the meat and juice are inside of us. I believe what my insiders say happened. The feelings and physical sensations my body experiences confirm these experiences no matter how awful they are to endure.

If you are suddenly in pain week after week, you might be being beaten up regularly. It pays to ask inside about that. If you are chronically ill, it pays to ask inside whether you have programming to be ill and incapacitated. That is how they slow many truth-seekers down.

The first step in becoming who you are is to believe in yourself. This will go against every bit of programming you ever had—programming to do things you would never choose to do and will feel ashamed of. Programmers make you think you deserve nothing from life and are only a marionette on a tight string, a means for others to get what they desire. They believe they have made you into a slave and servant exclusively. You are not who they made you think you are. You are good and worthwhile. You deserve to live and to be in the place on earth where you reside. If you are currently being accessed, you deserve to move far away from your perpetrators. You deserve the food you eat and the water you drink. You deserve.

You deserve to be you. You deserve to belong to yourself. You are yourself and yours alone—for better or worse and in recovery and freedom. You are worthwhile and essential.

Search your life for love. Did you have a friend who was kind? Was a sibling ever protective, appreciative? Did anyone ever acknowledge you—a teacher perhaps? If you cannot find anything but hatred, then look somewhere else. Were your parents ever reasonable or friendly, generous? If you still cannot find anything, then go into yourself. Were you ever good to yourself? If not, you can start now and this will be the foundation of learning about love. You are leaving the world of hatred and entering the realm of love: gentle, encouraging, respectful, caring. Memorize how it feels. People care about you. You care about you. Kindness to the self unhinges the mind control within the brain. You are not a bad person. Once the belief that you are a bad human being leaves, you are *en route* to dismantling mind control. Its foundation is self-hatred and the belief that you are unlovable. Those lies can be exposed. You are a worthwhile, moral human being who deserves to be alive and do good in the world. You are not a robot. You are not an automaton.

Here is an exercise: Take something about yourself that you do not appreciate and decide to love it—your nose, legs, hair, disposition, jealousy, anger, handwriting. Work on seeing its beauty, work on seeing it in a new light. This is just a preliminary exercise to help you re-evaluate yourself and give up what your programming wants you to believe about yourself. It is a step toward saying goodbye to self-hatred, false ideas, and lies.

List what you deserve in life, such as love, comfort, praise, encouragement. Now you are changing the self-esteem from the front person inward. It is the children within you who are convinced they are bad. But when the front people change their beliefs, it affects the whole internal system. It is like water coming through a hole in the roof and bathing the interior. Soon, even the self-hating small children can learn about self-love.

When you are in a tortured, unloved state, you will believe what you would not otherwise believe. Mind control begins on the innocent, the ones too small to think through the lies and preposterous statements, the visuals, and torture.

Here is another issue: Small internal children cannot understand tricks and lies. Their minds are not formed enough to understand manipulation. This is one reason why integration is necessary. When I reached these young parts, they could not understand all the visual and aural tricks my relatives and programmers played on me. They grappled and struggled with this dilemma but no matter how hard they tried, they just could not get it. They are bright children, but it was beyond them. The internal adults tried to explain the lies. No dice. When these darling, hard-working children eventually fused with older parts, their distress ended. Too much had been expected of them. Inside, they finally got to play games and do puzzles and read children's books, even after they fused. I still go to the library and take out children's books at least once a month. But the inside adults do the thinking. The child parts were subsumed into adulthood and in adulthood people can understand lies and tricks and evil and monstrosities. Adults might not have a strong stomach, but they can understand.

Once you understand the lies you live your life by, you can change. You can give up so much, including, and perhaps most importantly, how you feel about yourself. Forgiveness starts with the self. You can forgive yourself for what other people did to you. After integration, there might be a life review of things and actions you regret. This life review gives you the opportunity to forgive yourself for not being yourself, for not being a whole person capable of making wise decisions and treating others with utmost respect. You can forgive yourself for your past and how it shaped how you were in life. And now you can change.

When you finally get into recovery and after recovery, you look back on your life lived as a non-self. The sooner you start dismantling your programming, the fewer years you will have to regret having lived as a robot, slave, and non-self.

We manage, but it is hard to live with no true self. It is a testament to our endurance that we are alive. We now deserve the reward of finding out who we are. When I finally asked myself who I am for real, I discovered that I had been sent to, and temporarily submitted to, five planted therapists.

Much of what I thought I did on my own initiative was programmed in.

I had to look back on a life without choice.

But then someone, or ones in you, make the big decision and the earlier the better, but best at any time—just not never.

Start by distinguishing between programming and how you really feel about yourselves.

If you can, find a therapist who does not think the worst of you, who does not look down on you. Planted therapists will usually give some hint that they look down on you.

Ask your emotions "Who are you?"

Your emotions might answer that they are not allowed to have feelings, that no crying is allowed, that you cannot feel good about yourself. It is just about impossible to get over these traumatic feelings without doing something to release them, such as crying. Your programmers know that. When you start to cry, you have started to heal. For some, try crying instead of cutting yourself.

Programmers observe and figure out what is particularly repulsive to you and make you believe that about yourself. They want you to think the worst about yourself and it will not be true.

Once your self-esteem improves, your mind control will start to dismantle and dissolve and you will see changes in yourself. You will not be sent out to perform criminal deeds. You may start remembering what they wanted you to do. Those are the enormous changes. There are more subtle ones that affect your daily life. Before, every little mistake or flaw you perceived as large and interpreted as an indictment against yourself. With better self-esteem, you will see those mistakes as little mistakes and no big deal. They are highly correctable. Simply mistakes.

Once your self-esteem improves, you begin to parent yourself and take yourself through developmental stages. You become your own mother and father, the ones most of us never had.

If you have poor self-esteem, you care too much about what other people think of you. You were trained to do whatever your programmer and handler command. You are used to putting too much emphasis on another's opinion. With low self-esteem, you look hungrily at other people to determine who you are. As you get to know yourself, and all there is in you, you gain respect for yourself and begin to trust yourself. You are the ultimate authority on yourself. You do not have to ask other people's opinion about yourself. Once you believe in yourself, everything changes. You are no longer devastated if jerks do not like you or your work. If you are rejected, it does not crush you. You stand by yourself. No one can manage your life anymore. You become self-sufficient. You give up being family-hungry.

You will be able to tolerate change. No matter what you do, change will happen in your life. It happens in everyone's life. With low self-esteem, change can create a resistant paralysis in you. You will not be sure you can handle it. With improved self-esteem, you have the confidence to go with the flow and adapt to what you need to adapt to.

In addition to unraveling mind control and improving your self-esteem, here are more ways to encourage healing.

Take more moments enjoying hot water warming your back in the shower.

Savor fruit the way food was supposed to taste before chemicals and modern farming methods.

Find yourself seconds of pure, untampered-with pleasure. The skin's pleasures have been contaminated and corrupted all during your mind-controlled life. Now it is time to teach your skin what it means to be skin. The pleasure principle helps you find yourself. Enjoy a breeze, which can be better than a lover.

The breeze—where it coats your body with such gentleness, concern, and languor—brings you to the edge of life, makes you whole, offers you a fountain to drink from that belongs to everyone and no mind controller could ever take that away.

To shed the slave mentality, say:

I deserve . . .

I am . . . [and fill in the blanks].

Go deep within yourself to realize at last who you are.

It is better to find someone to share your memories with. That was important to me. If a safe person is not available, journal your insights and understandings and keep going alone.

The pool of emotions underneath

Wendy Hoffman

After you have delved and scratched and inched your way through mountains of programs held in parts, all of which are surrounded by episodes of torture, after you have finished most of this arduous work, you arrive at your base and may, amazingly enough, find pools of emotions held by yet other pieces, though off-shoots of parts you have already met. Even though you may have integrated your primary personalities, you could find that you have a half-healed heart. In this pool of emotions is a bottom layer of being that is you at a primitive emotional level.

The cult leaders' plan for you included controlling your emotional life. They began by breaking or preventing your bond with your mother. This created a loneliness that hurts even physically and can be life-threatening. This loneliness can make the heart spasm, limbs ache, stomach churn. It surrounds you as an infant with a cloud of hopelessness and takes away the desire to partake of life, thrive, and survive. It is a gruelling feeling. Young victims drag this emotional state throughout their childhoods, especially after the murder of their only designated friend. The stab of this loneliness can be unbearable. Each victim then goes through much of his or her unhealed life afraid to love and bond, wanting no one else to be murdered. No matter how severe the physical torture, the emotional torture that pierces innocence is the worst. The emotional foundation of not having bonded creates a strong, bleak fortress.

The loneliness that resides at the base of the newly born infant can last throughout life. Even after healing that includes the spontaneous melding together of parts of the brain, this loneliness can become a permanent fixture. Loneliness can follow even those survivors young enough to marry and create new families. Living with people can make one even lonelier. People are not usually aware of this loneliness. It is hidden deeply and flickers in and out of consciousness, sometimes seen, often missed.

Some can shed the loneliness drop by drop as they perfect their healing and enter into a life of their own choosing. Others become married to this primitive state and are dominated by the deprived infant parts their whole lives, trying unsuccessfully to care for them or find others who will. Some, in both the cult and non-cult worlds, cannot outgrow these early deprivations and carry around with them their internal small beings with unmet needs.

However you choose to deal with the physical and emotional pain of early infancy, it is better to know that it is there and to manage it. Some try to manage the pain by never being alone. The fear of being alone has led people into terrible arrangements, soul-crushing marriages, doing far too much for people who want to misuse you. Not knowing about your primitive loneliness can drive you into more usurping relationships.

Feelings can be a normal response to what is happening in your current life. Ask yourself which responses are appropriate responses to the present, and which are left over from the past (even if triggered by present events) and not yet fully connected to their original sources and discharged. It is particularly difficult and painful to go through infants' emotions, where everything is intense and immediate. Understanding yourself as an infant may help you grow into adulthood emotionally.

Another bottom-of-the-system feeling is shame. Shame is sometimes underneath the loneliness. Shame also has to be either released slowly or acknowledged and managed. Healed survivors can cognitively work through the lies that made them feel responsible and ashamed fairly easily. Most survivors have been forced to participate in the murder of the innocent. Perpetrators use the hands of child victims. Some survivors can see that they were not responsible for what others forced them to do when they were children. But others cannot overcome the shame of having been implicated in a crime that took away another's life. They wrestle with this shame and may experience it life-long, even though they would never have chosen to murder on their own.

In addition, as part of resolving shame, survivors have to deal with sexuality and their sexual responses. Survivors have been used as sexual objects, some as soon as they were born. These cults often combine death and sexuality. Even survivors who have come into their healings late in life will have to come to terms with their sexual being if they want to manage the shame instilled as early as that emotion can first be felt. People with relaxed, open bodies that they fully occupy have usually not been sexually abused. A body free of lifelong tension would be a goal for survivors of mind control who were used as sexual puppets. They can gradually learn to take pleasure in their bodies, to be in their own bodies. Start with touching any part of your own body, and practice not dissociating as you do this. Peel yourself off the ceiling and work on staying in your own body.

It is not surprising that buried in this submerged nest of emotion is rage. The rage is reasonable and understandable but it is gathered together here and is overly intense. Survivors are angry at the torture they endured from birth onward, that they could not be who they were meant to be, and that they had to run and hide from their previous lives. They are mostly angry at what they were made into and what they had to do. They are angry that they are different from the normal world and have trouble fitting in.

It does not help the raging person to scream at his or her pet or at an automated voice in customer service over the telephone. Then, what is there to do with the rage? Feel it, know it, acknowledge it. The rage is fitting for what happened then but too extreme for present circumstances. Let it leave the body drip by drip. This is the rage you could not express to your perpetrators as they tortured you. As you put a wall between the past and present and realize that the intense emotions belong back there, you will regain your equilibrium. Eventually, this invisible wall will not be needed and will crumble. The energy that comes with and from rage can be redirected to help society. For example, you can become an activist for human rights, or you can expose the reality of criminal mind control and ritual abuse and work towards stopping it.

Once you scrape off the intensity of rage, you might find depression. Why should you not be depressed? A life in these cults contradicts what life is meant to be. You observe people in ordinary life getting upset about things that are barely significant. You have important realities to be sad about. Appropriate sadness is not clinical depression and is not a mental illness. It is not to be medicated away.

Underneath the loneliness, shame, rage, and depression comes guilt. As my mother was dying in a Bronx hospital, she screamed out at me the rage that she had not had a life, and that I had ruined her image. I was her whipping girl. Whatever went wrong in her life she blamed on me. At the end, she said to me, "We had our moments." In these dark worlds, some only have moments of relating, of decency. Moments do not make a mother. I have always been motherless; someone else might have transcended the mind control somewhat, but she did not. She lived in an era when no help existed. The programmers knew that. Had she lived now, she may have broken free.

Once you realize the set-ups, guilt is not so hard to overcome. Cognitively, survivors can reason these false scenarios away and know that their blame is a giant lie. I do not accept responsibility for my mother's whole life, although she thought I should. Mind control procedures attempt to make victims feel that they are responsible for every bad thing that happened. The leaders want you to feel bad about yourself. You do not have to go through life with that false belief.

Even as rage and depression are connected, so are guilt and anxiety. The undercoating of survivors' lives is anxiety. Some of us grew up not knowing what would happen next, not knowing when our caregivers would switch into menacing, homicidal parents. Anxiety was a constant companion, present even when we were not aware of it. Anxiety is appropriate if you are still being hunted by perpetrators. But if you are one of those fortunate survivors who is actually safe in the present, the anxiety belongs to the past, and you can now learn to relax.

Slowly work your way through the remaining nest of feelings. Acknowledge the lies and threats that made you feel the way you do. Then create a life that does not twist your heart and keep you from your true self. You know who you are by your feelings. Clear out of your heart the intense emotions programmers put in you on purpose, which belong to the past, and replace them with emotions that do what they are intended to do, which is letting you know about whether or not your needs are met in the present.

When a program engulfs you

Wendy Hoffman

I believed I was the me I knew, the me who was pretty much finished with the excavations, the me who could think clearly, was compassionate, and was filled with sorrow about how the world is. But then a new me galloped out and, with narrowed eyes, reviewed the way in which significant people thought of me. I latched on to a fleeting look or glance to make a case that the person or people held me in low regard. I would think, "These people are glad to get rid of you, they are tired of you, they think you have no boundaries, you have exhausted them, you exhaust everyone."

I wondered why I was having these alienating thoughts. How come I was gripped at this late stage by the irrational and lies? Another program had emerged. I scraped and found something painful, shocking, and disappointing at the bottom of the barrel.

The public has read for years now how the Catholic church has been guilty of sexually abusing children and colluding with its perpetrators. This did not shock me. I wrote about being abused at a famous religious center in my memoir, *The Enslaved Queen* (2014). I knew that every religion has perpetrators and that they hide behind the prestige and respectability of religious office.

But I did not know that the revered rabbi with whom I had studied the Torah line by line was one of the leading torturers and programmers in the community I had lived in. And so were other esteemed rabbis in this same community. This rabbi, my teacher, founded a synagogue to bring people back to Judaism. The people I thought were my sincere friends were his assistant torturers. I felt as if I was hopping on melting ice. I could have been one of the sea animals whose whole habitat was dissolving.

My memory led me back to where this program about everyone despising me was put in. I am underground, below a landmark-like temple in this same community. There are spinning wheels to which people can be tied to disorientate them and make them too dizzy to function or think, particularly elaborate head vises, rows and rows of electroshock chairs. It must be a programming center. In my already healed mind, I had not known it existed. Many such places are all over the world. Pretend Judaism is the perfect cover for Nazi perpetrators.

This is what the rabbi said as he and others tortured me: "You bring trouble and despair everywhere you go. No one wants you around. You are danger, fire, a plague. You bring danger and destruction to everyone you know. You are a horrible person. We should rid the world of you. You are bad, you are awful . . ." My "friends" chanted these slogans. Drugs, electricity, all kinds of torture—the usual. This torture specialist enhanced some of Mengele's, the Nazi's, ideas. Mengele sometimes worked by torturing two victims simultaneously. The rabbi refined the method. Whip one victim, who was a frail, sick woman in this case, as someone else whips the other victim, me. Then Taser them simultaneously. I survived the torture. I was told my bad actions or thoughts—how could they know my thoughts?—had caused this disgrace.

The program barged out before the memory. The program caused paranoia. I sullied the innocent. I sullied myself. Discovering the memory brought me back to sanity. The periphery or wide margins of me engulfed the center and I returned to "normal." The healed mind overtook the programmed slice of mind.

How do you prevent programs from exploding? Get as many of the training memories out as possible. Expect particularly disheartening ones at the bottom of the barrel. Strengthen the periphery. The periphery is the part of you no longer programmed. You are a rational being. You can tell whom to trust. Listen to the knowledge you have acquired. When you are gripped against your will by urges or emotions you cannot stop, look for the memories that created them. After it is all done, be glad you will not be controlled by that stinking program again. This is the life of people who were formerly slaves.

I never suspected my "friends" were victims, too. They seemed so self-righteous. Do not underestimate how many people in your world could be cult. They are like flocks. Many people trying to get out are surrounded. The main danger comes from programs still within. When your feelings go crazy, look for programs that others put in you and that take you far away from yourself. When you find the programs and how they were installed, your sanity will return.

In the beginning years of therapy, either with a therapist or on your own doing self therapy, programs immediately jump out. Typical ones are kill yourself, do not believe what you remember, there is no such thing as dissociation or multiplicity, you do not have parts or alters, come back to us, bring this message here, contact that person there, attend a ritual at this date at this time at this location—instructions will follow, seduce him or her, steal this or that—for some, murder this person or that person, and so on. Inherent in all these programs is an assault on self-esteem. How could people be mindless marionettes and feel good about themselves? Even programs discovered late include an attack on self-esteem.

Here is more of what the rabbi said to me underneath the prestigious synagogue.

"You may never escape, you may never be free. We are your rulers, we are your enforcers, we are your kings, you are our property. Never go near anyone who tells you differently. You are our slave. We will put you in your grave. You have disobeyed us. You are finished."

That is how programmers talk as they torture.

As you remember these kinds of programs, you might realize that in the past you have driven away good people by distrusting their affection, and that you have ruined good opportunities for yourself. But along with that sadness is the joy that you are finally doing something about it. Even a day of freedom makes it worthwhile.

After I wrote about the abuse by the rabbi, I expressed to Alison that, in writing about this, I would endanger Jews all over the world. She pointed out that it did not endanger Catholics when survivors spoke out about priests; it made them safer. I continued to express my belief, and she told me that she thought I was "speaking from programming." I searched inside and found programming to make me believe that if I disclosed this abuse, there would be another Holocaust and all the Jews would be murdered.

"Speaking from programming" is something that Alison and I have been learning about over the course of our relationship. She is getting better at identifying it, and so am I. When I say something that is irrational and out of character, it is generally an indication that a program is operating. The same is true for other survivors. Therapists, if a survivor client is adamant about something that is clearly irrational, there is a good chance that he or she is speaking from programming. Do not argue with a program; you will not win. Just get down to business: it is an opportunity to identify the program and discover how it was made. Survivors, when words come out of your mouth that just do not make sense, find out which part of you is saying them, then search inside for when they were put in. These are giant steps to becoming who you are.

When you have killed*

Alison Miller

This is an account of a therapy session with child parts of an adult client, a survivor of organized mind control by a right-wing political group. The survivor's words (mostly coming from child parts) are in regular script (with odd words in italic for emphasis); the therapist's words are in italics, with some roman for emphasis. The language is childish because a very young part was speaking. The subject matter is a child being forced to kill. Only read it if you are ready to deal with this subject matter. The client does find considerable relief by the end of the session.

* * *

We all share so everybody knows that what the bad people do is not what we want to do. We're trying to get to the part where it upsets everybody if we hear a baby cry.

We're supposed to be a killer, nobody's gonna change that. It's who we are, it's in our DNA.

How old are you?

---

* A version of this chapter was published in the online journal, *Survivorship*, Winter 2016.

Five.

Do you know what DNA is?

No.

Is this a program?

It's a program. They have a baby over there, crying, and they bring another baby in. Every time, you see a baby crying and they bring in one that's still.

We are the sleepers. They're trying to reconstruct the nature of the person by repetition, over and over. It's important to get the senses. We have to keep our eyes open so we can see for real. You do not know who you are any more. You only have so much energy.

The program is unspinning . . .

Somebody inside would use the memory of the baby crying, while we stabbed. The live baby initially over on the left side, the still baby by us. Then later in rituals no live baby was needed. We never know if the baby we kill is alive or dead when we kill it. Sometimes in the early stages the body got electrocuted while the baby cried.

What were the instructions?

"Whenever the ritual starts you try to hear the baby crying." The body was three and a half when they said that. You're strapped to the table, hear crying, get electrocuted. Part of it was done in the hospital, then they continued in the church. You just see the baby and think he's crying and think there'll be electricity and the baby will get killed. The electricity was in the head. The arms and legs were strapped down. Jesus [the alter involved] is the immortal one and has power over life and death. The sleeper, who are also Jesus, have to go through it too. They are told to watch so when one Jesus fails there are still the sleepers. The sleepers stay on the outside of the body and watch. They take over. It's part of their job to come into the body.

All the sleepers, all the Jesuses need to join in as we go through the memory of these trainings.

They're just saying "Killer, killer, killer, killer . . ." They always say the Aryan race is superior, all hail the Aryan race, heil Hitler. They chant [gibberish]. They're making us killers to honour the Aryan race. That means the blond-haired blue-eyed ones like us. Jesus is the key, who gets raised from the dead. He has the power. Nobody can hurt Jesus because he's already dead. The Jesus that gets created is immortal.

None of you is immortal.

What is your left hand doing?

It's making a sign to make sure everybody in this memory is accounted for and present.

We have to drink the blood after, and eat the organs, because the power's in the blood that makes us have the power over life and death. And they keep making us do it till we do not flinch or get sick. "You're the killer, you do not think. We have the power, we can take your life." It's all for the purpose to make the ultimate killer.

When the body became ten they let go of the arm and it kept moving, it got caught up in the motion. "You're the killer. All hail the Aryan race." We wished the arm had kept moving and cut us up instead.

The boy's going to be killed anyways, and it'll be slower or worse if *they* do it than if we do it.

Who in you decided to let the arm keep moving and kill the boy without anyone's hand on yours?

Essence [the core spiritual essence] decided. Essence always knows the truth. It was a choice you should never have to make.

They always blamed us, and said we would go to hell. All these years we've been going crazy because of it.

Essence chose what would make the boy suffer least. You did not choose that *he would die, you only chose* how *he would die, the least painful way.*

So we're *not* evil! It was really a *kind* thing that we did. That's weird. We showed *mercy*. We thought we were going to eternal damnation.

We never thought we'd get this relief.

* * *

This was a very meaningful therapy session for the survivor. If you are a survivor reading about it, I hope it will help relieve your guilt and shame for your forced choices.

Giving up dissociation

Wendy Hoffman

Dissociation is one of the worst things that can happen to a life, even though it is the best thing that can occur during torture. Unfortunately, to find out about the torture, you have to give up dissociation. Those who are the most dissociated do not even know their dissociation exists. The way to find out is to have someone tell you.

When dissociation is gone, the thick black lines that hold the many parts of the brain distinct begin to smear, dissolve, and disappear. Blood suddenly runs through from one section to another. The brain may spasm, hiccup, get fuzzy and dizzy, but then the movement subsides and the mind becomes solid. Try shaking your head hard. It will not come apart. Your mind is now closer to how minds were designed to be before the interference and subterfuge.

What are the consequences of losing your dissociation?

You now have access to all feelings. Your emotions are no longer sectioned off into buried, distinct, hidden, long-suffering parts of the mind. The heart, once frozen, now bears the burden.

I never thought it would happen to me, but it has. Most of my brain is together now. If I twist my head hard, it still stays intact. If I bend it way to the right, it does not re-split. If I swing it to the left, most of me is still integrated. I find memories and emotional states still not known or raw inside me, but they are not dangling in their own world. They live in my melded and unified mind. I have given my mind the space and knowledge to unify.

Who am I now? I love myself. I am gentle and caring towards myself. I have trekked out of a lifetime of horrendous abuse, but I am whole now. I have inflated my crushed and flattened body, mind, and soul.

I used to avoid pain by splitting away when it arose. I could even split away from broken bones. One part of me would feel the pain but the rest would proceed with life as if nothing happened. Now, when I hurt, I hurt straight through.

The sting of emotional pain pierces. The emotions are shared throughout me, which means mature portions of me can consider and advise about this state of being. A whole movement of comforting myself sweeps over me now. I am my own best friend. I am my mother and father as well.

Integrating this late in life brings remorse and regret. Before, I believed the lies my controllers told me under torture—that my child would be tortured and slowly murdered, that this friend, that helper would have similar fates if I disobeyed. Instead of finding my own mind and running, I stayed trapped to protect other people. My "protecting" them did no good. Awareness of assumptions made by naïve child parts is part of the knowledge that takes place post-integration. I have to accept my stupidity and live with it. It does not pay to let it eat me up alive. A wave of self-forgiveness helps assuage the burning sting. All odds were against me. I had enemies. I did not have help. I did what I could.

Loneliness is another post-integration issue. When I meet a non-traumatized person from the normal world, I observe how that person lives and her character, and I face what I never had: a real life. Even some people who know about the abuses I suffered do not understand what it was like. I have experienced almost every kind of suffering and it has left me a have-not in a have-everything kind of world.

But I remember, and I have a soul and a conscience.

Is there an end to the healing process?

Wendy Hoffman

Some survivors may make huge progress during the beginning and middle periods of their recovery, have years of getting on with life in an ordinary way, and then new parts appear. That is how we know we have not finished recovery. This pattern may persist throughout a lifetime and raises certain questions. Should survivors be informed that locating and healing all parts of their mind-controlled brains may be a life-long endeavor and might never be fully accomplished? Should this information be part of informed consent? But would survivors then be discouraged from even beginning to dismantle their mind control? Would only the most earnest truth-seekers even try to be free? And would the already scarce therapists not want to go into the field? People like to finish what they start. And therapists do not want to be stuck with survivor-victims life-long. Success and an end point seem to be two necessary components of taking on work for some. Is it wrong, then, for a therapist to tell clients a process will end when it might not? It could also be wrong to tell clients the process might never end when it might end.

Since, to my knowledge, other survivors of mind control have not spoken about this, I will use my own experience as an example. After the year I spent in intensive therapy with Alison, I kept working on my own and found other traumas. Then I had a hiatus of relative peace during which I enjoyed nature. Eventually, I received an email with trigger words from one of the "friends" who lived in the city I escaped from and whom I thought of as a friend, at one time my best friend. I might never have gotten to this awareness and the related programming memories on my own. The reason the "friend" directed me to it is because it is a potent and complicated suicide program that the abusers wanted me to act on. When I was an older child, the infamous Mengele captured three of my original thirteen infant parts, bound them and locked them in an airtight internal chamber where they received no food or drink. He built on those death experiences through torture and programmed an older child to kill herself. I had missed this whole piece of my mind control, though I had remembered many other suicide programs, some installed by this same Nazi doctor. This awareness opened up the vital information about how many of my "friends" were cult plants.

Recently, I found internal structures within a structure. This is the internal structure that the Nazi group erected when they stole the parts that the Illuminati group created when I was born. There was a giant cave with a tower and smaller caves within the main cave. By its side was what Mengele called a red river. I worked through the contents of this structure and revived the stolen parts. Then I saw within my brain little *papier-mâché* and clay models and tarot cards. The red river became a piece of painted red cardboard. It is all just paper. There is the tower constructed of paper and clay. Toothpicks hold it up. Toothpicks, and I thought it was a prison. And there is the tarot card of a tower. A woman or girl falls out its window. She will land on a tiny table. The fall will not break her back. There were many cards of crows. Crows live for three years. Those crows cannot still be alive. What was erected was a paper world that comes down like a child's collapsible toy. This is a paper hell, a child's hell. The river is dry. Soggy playing cards remain at the bottom. The hearts, spades, clubs, diamonds are smeared with ink that has run. Soggy little playing cards that controlled me. This was an imaginary internal world within my child-brain. It is no longer real.

I do not know how many more devastating surprises I will find. Perhaps none, perhaps many. Only time will tell. Whether there is an end to discovering what criminal mind control you have been subjected to is something people have to hang loose about. I have the skills now to work through the new memories and programs to commit suicide, which will not affect me. I doubt fully that I am the only survivor who will find new chambers in my mind that I have not had the lucidity to get to earlier, despite an enormous effort. I do not know whether there is ever a true end to this process. I hope there is. If there is not, what freedom I have achieved will be enough.

Will there be an end to the world?

Will there be an end to restoring the split and chopped up mind?

Will there be an end to internal parts and parts held in reserve and parts stolen by one group from another?

Even experienced therapists can be shocked to learn how long it takes to treat survivors of generational criminal mind control. They may sign on for years and find they have to work with the same clients for decades. Naturally, they become impatient. Some become exhausted and want their lives back. Who would not? It is difficult to maintain a normal, carefree life while treating survivors. In addition, the helpers are forced to acknowledge what occurs in dark society and some do not want to see. Therefore, there may be an inherent, though unconscious, rushing in the treatment. They might silently encourage a belief that survivors have finished when, in fact, there is more work to be done. They might proclaim that there is an end to this kind of treatment, to the reunification of the once-split mind. For some, there might be. But for others, there might not be.

There can still be an end to therapy, however. Once you have worked with a skilled therapist for a while, you may have learned how to do the work yourself. People who have had an intensive course of "regular" therapy for traumas less intense and prolonged than mind control often go back for a check-up if symptoms start to reappear. You are allowed to do that, if your therapist is still available. You deserve it.

SECTION VIII

ODES ABOUT MIND CONTROL

by Wendy Hoffman

I wrote some of these Odes to reach out to the different parts of myself who have had horrendous jobs in their secret lives, and also for survivors who are looking within and finding tragedy. I hope the Odes offer compassion.

* * *

To the Mind-Controlled

You were born whole, lovely and good.
They tortured your brain into thousands of pieces.

You became many strangers,
each one living in an ice-concealed grave inside.

Hordes in ghostly isolation, not one knew of the others.
Noiseless, you tiptoed through life, alone in a mob.

I am happy that I did not stay in a shattered mind.
I followed the invisible thread back.

Let the pain flood into the Red Sea.
Nothing is worth sacrificing truth for. And freedom.

Nothing is worth not becoming yourself.

To the Front Person

You have lived your life in the one quarter inch of space
in my outer crust.
You did not know how the rest of us suffered within.

You walked down the sidewalk and up the hill as if you were like
everybody else.
You did not know you were empty and filled to bursting.

You smiled a normal smile which often came about suddenly.
People said you have a nice smile. That means you must be normal.

You went to school and day dreamed.
You did not know they put learning problems in you.
You passed anyway.

You married and divorced confused.
Why wasn't your husband a good man? Why didn't you get along
with your son?

You did not know about all the abducted children or your
murdered friend.
You did not know about your most important people.

You did not know you did not know.
You went through life not knowing a thing, much like society today.

How brave you were. Taking steps forward, not knowing you carried
frozen hordes within.
You felt their emotions but could not name them.

You did not understand that you were empty and over-full to bursting.
How valiant to get an education and paid work, to move forward not
knowing you were empty and over-full.

You shoveled snow off the deck, worked two jobs, sometimes
 were kind.
You slogged through life, had moments of buoyancy.

And when you broke down and could no longer do it, they
 created another front person.
And still you did not know. Then you were inside among the silent.

How valiant and brave and sad.
And now you know. You are the over-full. You name the feelings.

Unlike society, you understand.
How valiant and brave and sad.

*To the Unloved, Rejected and Abandoned**

It wasn't your fault.
Right from the start, we were emptied out
 and raw hatred inserted.
They trained our mothers to turn their backs on us,
 our fathers to be brutal.
Your grandfather may be your father.
How could your mother overcome that?
 Our heritage.
It is your mission now to love yourself.
You are as lovable as
 anyone else on earth.
You deserve to be cherished, not blamed.

To the Learning Disabled

Your mind drifted mid-sentence.
You could never finish a book.
You reversed letters and numbers.
Your mind inserted a 'not' in every sentence
and you stopped listening after a few minutes.

Teachers looked at you
with annoyance or pity.
You are stupid and dull—the only conclusion.

---

* A version of this poem appeared in the online journal *Survivorship*, Winter 2016.

Even your big sister said so, and she knew everything
and could read whole books.

But in college you heard whispers and dropped
comments that you have the smarts.
In graduate school the whispers
became more pronounced.

An optometrist detected your eyes muscles did not converge.
The vision trainer said it was caused by early loss.
Decades passed before you learned about mind control,
the government's secret.
Slaves always have to be rendered stupid.

More decades passed. In therapy
you remembered that before first grade,
programmers taught you not to read, not to do math, to give
wrong answers. To give a wrong answer, you first have to
figure out the right answer.

They buried your brightness under layers of weighted ineptitude.
Only they could use your intelligence, not you or any safe person.

To Spies, Thieves, and Mules

You learned to follow with soft steps, watch shadows, identify
people by their backs,
use your mind like a camera—snap, click, memorized.

You slipped documents and photos inside lapels and papers
out of inner pockets all while smiling sweetly and looking
sideways.

They shipped you around the world in an airplane seat or crate.
I got the information. I did the deed. I can go home.

The mules carried you to the criminal base you call home. They
managed Customs, read flight numbers. Each group had skills
they were not allowed to share with their companion-groups.
Without the mules, you would have remained in airspace.

Now airplanes and airports harrow. You do not have
to fly anymore.
You can stay home and use your nimble fingers digging in the
garden's earth and forming papier mâché shapes. No one will
send you off. Sit in the easy chair. Turn on the TV.

Even if you broke the mold and reported to Customs what you stole
or carried in your vagina, they would not have believed you.
You would have ended up with the "insane", drugged for life.

To the Sexual Slaves Within

I see a child on the stage as the brothel customers throw their wet
handkerchiefs at you. The spot lights hurt your body.

I see another child in the apartment building's basement learning
to fondle.
Uncle Mike taught you.

As a teenager in spiked heels, you slipped pills into drinks. Mengele
taught you.

You seduced and stripped on command. They have schools to teach that.
They separated many of you from the others. They wore one skin and
you grew a second skin of shame. People have died over less.

You had one of the harder jobs and you did not die even though
you died,
and died again.

Now you live with all of us in a solid globbing whole.

No one scorns you.
You do not have to be touched and you do not have to touch ever again.

A jewel in a velvet box, you are protected from the sinister.
You do not have to like men.
The others will take care of you.

Rest.
Here eat some chocolate.

To Mothers

So young. You gave birth before you were allowed to wear lipstick
in ordinary life.
They induced menstruation when you were eleven. And shipped
you off immediately to the Bronx brothel where your child's
body delivered three infants, immediately snatched away by
the Mafia adoption agency—to be sold like cocaine. You will
never see them. You couldn't hold or smell them. You do feel
them. You think your son is in jail. In the 1950s, other girls
starting junior high weren't allowed to date.

After thirteen, it was the Illuminati's turn. In a Brooklyn monastery,
you birthed
four more infants. You saw two murdered and do not know what
became of the others.
You grew an extra layer of skin inside your outer skin, a skin of
grief. You hold out your air arms and call your babies in. They fit
even though they are past middle age now. Did the slaughtered
infants stay infants? You press them to your heart and
your grief braids with theirs. Your and their angers clasp. Will you
see them in the afterlife? Is there an afterlife? You swim in air-reality.

To Kidnappers

Their goal is to strip you of all remnants of your real self.
You have to be an automaton who follows verbal, hand, foot

and visual signals.
They pull a string and the marionette moves.

That is what they make you.
They measure what would be most abhorrent to you.

Out of meanness or pleasure in their craft, they give you those tasks.
They are proud they have striped all your empathy away

but they cannot. Your own children were abducted
and you will always feel for children and mothers.

And so you have a screaming breakdown, exactly what
they do not want.

They try again years later.
They insist on perfecting evil.

You will keep living though so many children are dead.
You go on even though children are missing.

You did the best you could. "Under the worst circumstances"
has new meaning.

To Trained Assassins

You started out a meek and gentle soul.
But you could be quick to anger, the commanders noticed.
Their army needs killers:
because they have to kill
because they have to make you feel worthless.

Males have to go in with guns and fists.
Females learn seduction, pills and poisons.
Hefty girls can train with guns.
Stocky females with strong forearms become torturers too.

O, assassins, it is not who you are. You are still
innocent children sitting in a field of daisies.

They made you explode with anger. Drugs can do that.
They made you cold, calculating.

Come back to the beginning.
You have left behind the rest.
They took the sweetest part of you and twisted.

To Witches

Of all the jobs, this is not one of the worst.
You could travel on the periphery of breeze and wave,
cover vast terrains while gazing out your window.

You could be assigned to destroy but they do not know when
  you do the opposite. Maybe just the top experts would.

You didn't ask to be a witch or know how to make portents and charms.
You didn't ask to stroll into the future.

It doesn't matter.
Of course it matters.

To the Plant-Therapists

I cannot believe you would have done this of your own free will,
wittingly blocked people's paths,

cemented over their quest, made them about-face
in their belief in themselves. Some of you may be that evil.

But for the rest. You must have been badly tortured.
What was the threat? That your child would be murdered?

Worse?
That they would be skinned first?

Is your own child more important than other people's?
You took yearning minds and smashed them anew.

To Those Who Couldn't Protect

Bambi wasn't my dog though they bought him on my birthday.
  He was Father's dog.
He trained him.

At the Tackenasee country club, Mother held him by his hind legs
and beat him against the hotel's bathtub as if he were a dusty rug.
Father threw him in the swimming pool. Then Bambi bit a woman.
My parents.

When I was thirteen, Pow Wow attached himself to me. He became
the owner and
I the adored pet. He protected me until the commanders skinned
and sacrificed him.
My penalty for love.

Today my pet and I live in harmony, as peers.
But my front person was nowhere present when the tormenters
ripped into my home and twisted her back legs two different times.
A warning.

My front person thought the injury was genetic and rehabilitated
her all these years
but Blossom knew the truth.

How do you live with yourself when you couldn't protect?
You take one step, another and . . .

To the Beaten

Every month, in childhood every week, you were broken.

Right before I escaped, ruffians snuck through the back door, used
their key in the
front door, climbed my stairs and dragged, hit, tasered, raped and
plunged
me in a tub of ice.

That last day when I ran successfully, did they not know or were they
afraid of exposure? Is that why they let me go?

Unless they planned to murder me on the road.
Unless the friend who volunteered to accompany me is one of them.

Two and a half years later, my body softens. My toenails breathe.
I begin to
feel my bones grow sturdy, the hair on my arms, the ocean in
my nostrils.

You took the beatings for us all. You are sore and chipped.

Lie down in this hammock. Let the sun languish on your crushed
limbs, rock
back and forth, mend quietly.

You are free, safe and no longer numb.

To Mourners

Some people get over things. Some do not.

You have liquid skin and pliant muscles that should breathe out misery but you hold on.

You would be a different person today had he not loved you.

He was tall and thin with blue black curly hair that glistened in the dull air against his apricot skin and dark ancestral eyes. He was thirteen and he loved. You were three and a half.

Always, for sixty-nine years, you feel his breath on you, his heart beating upon yours, the rhythm of his lungs.

Take a child who knew only hatred and the gift of a boy who could only give love—take that and try to stop mourning.

To the Co-Conscious

In some ways, it was easier when everyone lived in their separate boxes.

The lids opened and thousands emerged, each with a story that would overwhelm any life.

Your old brain spasmed. Clogged pathways spit out rusted debris. Blood flowed to closed down cells. Your brain erupted into life. Springtime grew in snow and ice.

Eventually your brain quiets. All these people inside talk to one another. What conversations! You had no idea.

I believe it is better to know.
I believe truth is the goal.
But I had no idea.

To the Integrated

If I put my right ear to my shoulder, my mind still stays whole and fastened. If I tilt to the other side, I do not lose any parts.

I can move my head up and down, see the sky, earth—
it still all stays bound and backstitched.
I have had recent tragedies but my brain remains glued.
I hadn't even aimed for this cohesiveness. It happened by itself.

Emotions ripple through me.
All of me feels everything.
There is no escape from me.

All these pieces have come together to make me as close
to normal as a previously tortured person can become.
My mind walks toward how it was originally designed.
My heart has quadrupled.
I live inside my body.
My bones support me.

I move to the left, back, forward.
I stay intact.
My brain is having a reunion.

To Confidence

I have taken tiny steps—toe to heel—
around a lopsided globe

and flown upside down through the
circumference of wild air

but only now have I landed
among bones, organs and blood.

I have never been this close in myself before.
My new skin holds tightly as

I deliver bouquets,
truffles and creams to my arteries and veins.

It has been a long, tiring trip.
I rest quietly on the greenest prairie.

To Gratitude

My fingers are nimble
even though the tip
of one was amputated.

My teeth still chew
despite many socks
to the jaw.

My nostrils still sniff
despite the odor of
mounds of death.

My brain thinks
even though I have had more
concussions than football players.

I have come out alive
and can love.
That's enough.

REFERENCES

Carter, C. (2012). *Science and Psychic Phenomena: The Fall of the House of Skeptics*. Rochester, VT: Inner Traditions.

Extreme Abuse Survey (n.d.). Available at: https://eassurvey.wordpress.com/extreme-abuse-survey-final-results/.

Hoffman, W. (2014). *The Enslaved Queen: A Memoir about Electricity and Mind Control*. London: Karnac.

Hoffman, W. (2016a). *White Witch in a Black Robe: A True Story about Mind Control*. London: Karnac.

Hoffman, W. (2016b). *Forceps, Poems about the Birth of the Self*. London: Karnac.

Miller, A. (1983). *For Your Own Good*, H. Hannum & H. Hannum (Trans.). New York: Farrar, Straus, & Giroux.

Miller, A. (1997). *The Drama of the Gifted Child*, R. Ward (Trans.). New York: Basic Books.

Miller, A. (2011). *Healing the Unimaginable: Treating Ritual Abuse and Mind Control*. London: Karnac.

Miller, A. (2014). *Becoming Yourself: Overcoming Mind Control and Ritual Abuse*. London: Karnac.

Siegel, D. J. (2012). *The Developing Mind: How Relationships and the Brain Interact to Shape Who We Are* (2nd edn). New York: Guilford Press.

Woolston, C. (n.d.). Falling in love with your baby: the science behind love and mother–infant bonding. Available at: https://consumer.healthday.com/encyclopedia/parenting-31/parenting-health-news-525/falling-in-love-with-your-baby-643058.html.

INDEX

19792878R00179

Printed in Great Britain
by Amazon